Bayesian Biostatistics and Diagnostic Medicine

Bayesian Biostatistics and Diagnostic Medicine

Lyle D. Broemeling
The University of Texas
MD Anderson Cancer Center
Houston, Texas, U.S.A.

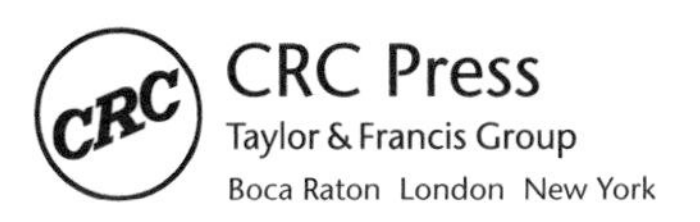

CRC Press is an imprint of the
Taylor & Francis Group, an **informa** business
A CHAPMAN & HALL BOOK

Chapman & Hall/CRC
Taylor & Francis Group
6000 Broken Sound Parkway NW, Suite 300
Boca Raton, FL 33487-2742

First issued in paperback 2022

ISBN 13: 978-1-03-247783-1 (pbk)
ISBN 13: 978-1-58488-767-6 (hbk)

DOI: 10.1201/9781584887683

Publisher's Note
The publisher has gone to great lengths to ensure the quality of this reprint but points out that some imperfections in the original copies may be apparent.

Library of Congress Cataloging-in-Publication Data

Broemeling, Lyle D., 1939-
Bayesian biostatistics and diagnostic medicine / Lyle David Broemeling.
p. ; cm.
Includes bibliographical references and index.
ISBN-13: 978-1-58488-767-6 (alk. paper)
ISBN-10: 1-58488-767-2 (alk. paper)
1. Bayesian statistical decision theory. 2. Diagnosis--Mathematical models. 3. Medicine--Research--Statistical methods. I. Title.
[DNLM: 1. Bayes Theorem. 2. Diagnostic Techniques and Procedures. 3. Data Interpretation, Statistical. WB 141 B865b 2007]

R853.S7B75 2007
610.1'519542--dc22 2006100996

Visit the Taylor & Francis Web site at
http://www.taylorandfrancis.com

and the CRC Press Web site at
http://www.crcpress.com

Table of Contents

Preface

Bayesian methods are being used more often than ever before in biology and medicine. For example, at the University of Texas MD Anderson Cancer Center, Bayesian sequential stopping rules routinely are used for the design of clinical trials. This book is based on the author's experience working with a variety of researchers, including radiologists, pathologists, and medical oncologists. The majority of that experience has been with the Division of Diagnostic Imaging, where radiologists determine the extent of disease among patients undergoing treatment. Diagnosis, via medical imaging, is essential in order to assess the effect of the various therapies provided to the patient. Another source of information for the author has been the ability to work with medical oncologists in their design of Phase I, II, and III clinical trials. The author has found Bayesian methods for the design and analysis of clinical trials to be quite useful because prior information, in the form of previous related studies, is always available and easily incorporated into the design of future studies.

Based on this experience and the wealth of information available to the author, this book should give the biostatistics student a good idea of what to expect and how to work with healthcare researchers. It is an introductory book with a Bayesian flavor and is directed toward diagnostic medicine. Students with a good background in the basic methods courses of regression and the analysis of variance and in the introductory courses in probability and mathematical statistics should benefit greatly from the book. With this type of background, the student will be able to learn Bayesian statistics and how to apply it to important problems in medicine and biology. In addition, it should serve as a useful reference for those providing statistical assistance to medical scientists.

In the book, the reader is introduced to various diagnostic medical procedures, then presented with the fundamentals of Bayesian statistics and associated computing methods. Next, the foundation for the analysis of diagnostic test accuracy is outlined and the Bayesian way to analyze such data is explained, using many author-assisted studies. Of special interest is the estimation of the area under the receiver operating characteristic (ROC) curve for determining diagnostic accuracy. Also described in the book is a novel way to estimate the area when the image data are clustered.

Some of the material in this book is similar to that found in *Statistical Methods in Diagnostic Medicine* by Zhou, Obuchowski, and McClish and *The Statistical Evaluation of Medical Tests for Classification and Prediction* by Pepe. Several examples from these sources are analyzed from a Bayesian perspective. However, this book is entirely from a Bayesian perspective and presents a great deal of material not stressed in the above-mentioned references. This material includes Bayesian methods of agreement between readers and the role diagnostic medicine plays in the design of clinical trials, and should complement as well as expand on the books by Pepe and by Zhou et al. A unique feature of this book is that the Minitab® and WinBUGS® packages are employed to provide Bayesian inferences. After reading the book, the student will be able to provide a Bayesian analysis for a large variety of interesting and practical problems.

Acknowledgments

The author would like to acknowledge the many departments and people at the University of Texas MD Anderson Cancer Center in Houston who assisted me during the writing of this book. First and foremost, I would like to thank the faculty in the Division of Diagnostic Imaging, who shared their valuable research expertise with me. Many of the examples of this book are a result of consulting with the radiologists in that division. In particular, Drs. Isis Gayed, Reggie Munden, Vikas Kundra, Edith Marom, and Sanjay Gupta are gratefully acknowledged.

Also, I would like to thank many people in the Department of Biostatistics and Applied Mathematics for the opportunity to be part of a developing biostatistics program. The assistance of the department in the areas of protocol development, the editorial services of Margaret Newell, and the programming assistance for Bayesian statistical methods were invaluable.

The National Cancer Institute awarded (1 P50 CA09345901 A1(PC-C)) Melanoma Spore to the UT MD Anderson Cancer Center (Dr. Elizabeth Grimm, principal investigator), and this provided support during the past 3 years.

Lastly, I want to give special thanks to my wife, Ana L. Broemeling, who always encouraged me during the many months of writing this book.

Author

Lyle D. Broemeling, Ph.D., is a research professor in the Department of Biostatistics and Applied Mathematics at the University of Texas MD Anderson Cancer Center in Houston. He received his B.A., M.S., and Ph.D. degrees from Texas A&M University at College Station. Since 1987, he has been active in consulting with medical researchers at the University of Texas Medical Branch in Galveston, the University of Texas School of Public Health, and the University of Texas MD Anderson Cancer Center in Houston. Dr. Broemeling's main interest is in developing Bayesian statistical methods and his previous books include *Bayesian Analysis of Linear Models* and *Econometrics and Structural Change*, written with Dr. Hiroki Tsurumi, Professor of Economics, Rutgers University.

Chapter 1

Introduction

1.1 Introduction

This book is about how to use Bayesian statistical methods to design and analyze studies involving diagnostic medicine. It grew out of the author's experience in consulting with many investigators of the Division of Diagnostic Imaging at The University of Texas MD Anderson Cancer Center (MDACC) in Houston. In a modern medical center, diagnostic imaging is ubiquitous and crucial for patient management, from the initial diagnosis to assessing the extent of disease as the patient is being treated.

1.2 Statistical Methods in Diagnostic Medicine

Biostatistics plays a pivotal role in the imaging literature, as can be discerned by reading articles in the mainline journals, such as *Academic Radiology, The American Journal of Roentgenology,* and *Radiology,* and the more specialized, such as *The Journal of Computed Assisted Tomography, The Journal of Magnetic Resonance Imaging, The Journal of Nuclear Medicine,* and *Ultrasound in Medicine.* As we will see, the usual methods ranging from the t-test and chi-squared test to others, such as the analysis of variance and various regression techniques, are standard fare for medical diagnostic studies. There are also some methods that are somewhat unique to the field, including ways to estimate diagnostic test accuracy and methods to measure the agreement between imaging modalities and/or readers. Also important to imaging research are the elements of good statistical design, including replication, randomization, and blocking in the planning of clinical investigations.

Diagnostic imaging is employed in clinical trials, such as Phase II trials, where the main objective is to determine the response to a new therapy and where the response is based on an image measurement. Patient sample size, based on Bayesian sequential stopping rules, is another application that has proven to be quite beneficial in the development of new medical therapies.

The Bayesian approach will be used throughout this book for all aspects of the design and analysis of diagnostic studies. Also, standard non-Bayesian methods will be employed on certain occasions when deemed appropriate.

1.3 Preview of Book

Chapter 2 is an introduction to the fundamental areas of interest in diagnostic medicine, including a brief description of the main imaging modalities, namely X-ray, computed tomography, magnetic resonance imaging, and nuclear medicine procedures. A brief explanation of how diagnostic imaging is involved in large population screening and in the day-to-day patient management is provided. The estimation of diagnostic accuracy is not only essential to the diagnosis of a patient, but also for the assessment of patient progress during therapy. Estimating agreement between various readers and/or modalities is crucial for the training of radiologists, for comparing imaging techniques, and in assessing the success of therapy. The development of an imaging modality involves three phases (Phase I, Phase II, and Phase III developmental trials) and these will be explained along with numerous examples. A description of the role diagnostic imaging plays in the various phases of a clinical trail is provided. In addition, the literature of the field, including the various books and journals, is reviewed.

The purpose of Chapter 3 is to introduce the reader to other areas of diagnostic medicine. In addition to diagnostic imaging, there are many other services that provide diagnostic information, including pathology and surgery. For example, in the treatment of breast cancer, it is imperative to know the extent of metastasis to the axillary lymph nodes. Sentinel lymph node (SLN) biopsies are performed to determine if there is lymph node involvement, and diagnostic imaging (including nuclear medicine and interventional radiology), pathology, and surgery are key components for the procedure. This chapter will examine the role of SLN biopsy in lung cancer and in melanoma. Of course, the biostatistical methods for determining accuracy and agreement are the same as those for diagnostic imaging, and their application to nonimaging tests will be shown.

Chapter 4 provides an introduction to Bayesian statistics, beginning with Bayes theorem and how prior information is found and used. Inferential techniques of estimation and testing hypotheses based on the posterior and predictive distributions are introduced. Also, how they are to be applied in diagnostic imaging is revealed. The computing algorithms along with the corresponding software for direct and indirect sampling from posterior distributions are briefly outlined. This book is unique in that the sample sizes are to be determined by fully Bayesian techniques, and the software that is used to estimate the sample size is described. Some of the packages are off–the-shelf, while others have been developed at MDACC.

Chapter 5 introduces the estimation of accuracy by sensitivity, specificity, and positive and negative predictive values for ordinal and continuous diagnostic measurements. Numerous examples taken from the literature illustrate the various concepts involved in test accuracy. The area under the receive operating characteristic (ROC) curve gives the overall intrinsic accuracy of an imaging modality, and Bayesian techniques that estimate this area are explained for ordinal and continuous data. Special software for Bayesian ROC analysis is introduced and illustrated with several examples analyzed by the author at MDACC. Also discussed are some specialized topics in test accuracy, such as problems of localization and detection, where multiple images are taken per patient. This induces a correlation between images within patients and special methods that take into account that correlation. The last topic of the chapter is on Bayesian sample size estimation for diagnostic accuracy.

In Chapter 6, the topics on diagnostic accuracy explained in the previous chapter are generalized to include patient covariate information. We know that test accuracy depends on many factors including patient characteristics, such as age, gender, therapy received, other biomarkers, stage of disease, etc. The importance of the risk score when taking into account patient covariates is emphasized and illustrated with many examples. Again, examples are based on the author's consultation with investigators in the imaging division of MDACC.

Often, the clinical investigator wants to know the extent of agreement between several readers or observers who are making diagnostic decisions. For example, one study at MDACC consisted of five readers estimating the size of a lung cancer lesion at various times in response to therapy. It is important to know the inter- and intra-observer agreement because it has a bearing on the decision to declare a therapy a success or a failure. Or suppose several readers are using a confidence level ordinal score to classify the status of lesions seen on a mammogram of a screening trial for breast cancer. How well do the readers agree? Chapter 7 discusses the statistical methods for estimating the agreement between and within observers, including a Bayesian version of the Kappa statistic to estimate agreement with ordinal data; for continuous data, regression techniques (including a Bayesian version of Bland-Altman) for calibration will estimate the agreement. In another example, three readers, reading the same image, measure the length and width of the major axis of spicules observed on mammograms. To measure inter-observer variability, analysis of variance methods, using random effects for readers and patients, calculate the agreement via the intra-class correlation coefficient.

Imaging techniques are utilized to measure the extent of response to therapy. For example, in many Phase II clinical trails for disease with solid tumors, the efficacy of the therapy is measured by the change in the size of the lesion from start of treatment. Imaging the tumor size is crucial. Chapter 8 provides the necessary detail in explaining the protocol review process for cancer clinical trials, how the tumor response is categorized, using World

Health Organization (WHO) and response evaluation criteria in solid tumors (RECIST) criteria, and lastly how Bayesian sequential methods are employed to monitor the trial and to estimate the sample size. Also discussed is the software development of Bayesian methods for the design and analysis of clinical trials at MDACC. Examples taken from the protocol review at MDACC illustrate how to apply Bayesian methods to this important application of diagnostic medicine.

Chapter 9 introduces other topics in diagnostic medicine that are not considered in the previous eight chapters. For example, how is the accuracy of a test estimated when there is no reliable gold standard, or how is accuracy estimated when only those that test positive are subject to the gold standard? Or suppose the gold standard is not binary, but is possibly continuous, then how is accuracy to be determined? Thus, this chapter emphasizes topics that do not fit the standard mold, but are variations of the basic themes introduced in the previous chapters. Other areas of medicine in addition to diagnostic imaging employ diagnostic tests for the management of the patient. For example, the whole idea of biomarkers, including the expanding area of genetic microarrays, is to use such information for medical diagnoses or as prognostic factors for patient morbidity and survival.

1.4 Datasets for the Book

The datasets used for this book come from the following sources: (1) the protocol review process of clinical trials at MDACC, where the author was either a reviewer or a collaborator on the protocol; (2) the author's consultations with the scientific and clinical faculty of the Division of Diagnostic Imaging at MDACC with some 32 datasets; (3) the six datasets accompanying the excellent book by M. S. Pepe[1] (see: http//www.fhcrc.org/labs/pepe/Book) *The Statistical Evaluation of Medical Tests for Classification and Prediction*; (4) the information contained in the examples of the WinBUGS® package; and (5) other miscellaneous sources, including the examples and problems in *Statistical Methods in Diagnostic Medicine* by Zhou, McClish, and Obuchowski.[2] Also, various articles by N. A. Obuchowski appearing in *The American Journal of Roentgenology* and *Academic Radiology* provided the author with useful information for this book, and several of her examples are included.

1.5 Software

WinBUGS will be used for the Bayesian analysis when sampling from the posterior distribution is appropriate. On the other hand, when direct sampling from the posterior distribution is called for, Minitab® is often employed for the posterior analysis. Many specialized Bayesian programs for the design and analysis of clinical trials have been developed at the Department of Biostatistics and Applied Mathematics at MDACC, some of which will be used for the design of clinical trials.

Why is the Bayesian approach taken here? The author has been a Bayesian theorist since 1974, when he was on a sabbatical leave to study at University College London. A colleague persuaded him of the advantages of such an approach. The main advantage, of course, is that it is a practical way to utilize prior information, which, in a medical setting, is all around and should be used to one's advantage. It would be a pity not to use it.

References

1. Pepe, M.S., The Statistical Evaluation of Medical Tests for Classification and Prediction, Oxford University Press, 2003, Oxford, U.K.
2. Zhou, H.H., McClish, D.K., and Obuchowski, N.A., Statistical Methods for Diagnostic Medicine, John Wiley & Sons, 2002, New York.

Chapter 2

Diagnostic Medicine

2.1 Introduction

In this chapter is a brief description of diagnostic imaging and other diagnostic techniques routinely used at a major healthcare institution. At MD Anderson Cancer Center (MDACC), the Division of Diagnostic Imaging is made up of the following departments: Diagnostic Radiology, Experimental Diagnostic Imaging, Imaging Physics, Nuclear Medicine, and Interventional Radiology. There were approximately 100 faculty members during the 2003–2004 academic year. Diagnostic imaging provides an extremely important role in the overall care of the cancer patient, including diagnosis, staging, and monitoring of patients during their stay in the hospital. Most of the examples in this book are taken from diagnostic imaging studies; however, there are many other ways to perform diagnoses, and some of these are explained in Chapter 3.

2.2 Imaging Modalities

The primary modalities for diagnostic imaging are X-ray, fluoroscopy, mammography, computer tomography (CT), ultrasonography (US), magnetic resonance imaging (MRI), and nuclear medicine. Each one has advantages and disadvantages with regard to image quality, depending on the particular clinical situation. Broadly speaking, image quality consists of three components. The first is contrast. Contrast is good when important physical differences in anatomy and tissue are displayed with corresponding different shades of gray levels. The ability to display fine detail is another important aspect of image quality and is called resolution. Anything that interferes with image quality is referred to as noise, which is the third component. Obviously, noise needs to be minimized in order to improve image quality.

Medical images are best thought of as being produced by tracking certain probes as they pass through the body. A stream of X-rays is passed through the patient and captured on film as the stream exits. An X-ray is a stream of photons, which are discrete packets of energy. As they pass through the body, various tissues interact with the photons and these collisions remove and scatter some of the photons. The various tissues reduce the amount of energy in various parts of the stream by different amounts. A shadow is produced that appears on special photographic film producing an image. If the density of the object that is the target is much higher than that of the surrounding environment (as bone), the X-ray does a good job of locating it. Some lesions have densities that are quite similar to the surrounding medium and are difficult to detect. Generally speaking, the X-ray has very good resolution and the noise is easy to control, but has low contrast in certain cases. The X-ray is routine in all medical settings and is the most utilized of all imaging devices.

A close relative of the X-ray is fluoroscopy. In this modality, the exiting beam is processed further by projecting it onto an image intensifier, which is a vacuum tube that transforms the X-ray shadow onto an optical image. This mode has about the same image quality as the X-ray, but allows the radiologist to manage images in real time. For example, it allows the operator to visualize the movement of a contrast agent past certain landmark locations in the gastrointestinal (GI) tract or vascular system.

Still another variation of the X-ray is computer tomography or CT, which overcomes some of the limitations of X-rays. The superimposition of shadows of overlapping tissues and other anatomical structures often obscure detail in the image. CT does produce images quite differently than X-rays; however it does use X-rays, but the detection and processing of the shadows is quite sophisticated and is the distinctive feature of the modality that vastly improves the image over that of the X-ray. CT has good contrast among the soft tissues (e.g., lung and brain tissue) and good resolution. The X-ray takes information from a three-dimensional structure and projects it onto a two-dimensional image, which causes the loss of detail due to overlapping tissues. To overcome this problem, the patient is placed in a circle and inside the circle is an X-ray source and embedded in the circle is an array of detectors that capture the shadow of the X-ray beam. The X-ray source irradiates a thin slice of tissue across the patient and the detector captures the shadow. The X-ray source moves to a close adjacent location and the process is repeated, say, 700 times. The X-ray source circumscribes the patient through 360 degrees. The source then repeats the above process with another thin slice. For a given slice, there are 700 projections of that slice and these 700 projections are processed via computer and back projection algorithms to produce the two-dimensional representation. The computer works backward from the projections to reconstruct the spatial distribution of the structure of the thin slice. In other words, CT answers the following question: What does the original structure need to resemble in order to produce the 700 generated projections?

A good example of CT (using the GE Imatron C-100 Ultrafast) is screening for coronary heart disease, where the coronary artery calcium score indicates the degree of disease severity. See Mielke et al.[1-3] and Dasgupta[4] where the accuracy of coronary artery calcium to diagnose heart disease is estimated by the area under the receiving operating characteristic (ROC) curve. These examples will be examined from a Bayesian perspective in later chapters.

Mammography is still another variation of the X-ray. While some small masses can be detected by a physician or by self-examination, mammography has the ability to detect very small lesions. However, the smaller they are the more difficult they are to detect. Mammography consists of a specialized X-ray tube and generator, a breast compression device, an antiscatter grid, and film. The procedure must be able to reveal small differences in breast density, possibly indicative of suspicious mass, and it must also be able to detect small calcifications that may have importance for diagnosis. All the attributes of good image quality are required, namely high contrast, good resolution, and low noise. Later in this book, the role of mammography in screening for breast cancer will be described.

A completely different form of imaging is magnetic resonance imaging (MRI). A beam of photons is not passed through the body, but instead the body is placed in a large magnet and the hydrogen atoms (in the water molecules) line up in the same direction as the magnetic field. When the magnetic field is disrupted by directing radio energy into the field, the magnetic orientation of the hydrogen atoms is disrupted. The radio source is switched off and the magnetic orientation of the hydrogen atoms returns to the original state. The manner (referred to as T1 and T2 relaxation times) and way in which they return to the original state produces the image. Essentially, what is being measured is the proton density per unit volume of imaged material. The actual image looks like an X-ray; however the principal foundations of MRI are completely different. The same image processing technology as used in CT can be used in MRI to process the images. For example, thin slices and backward projection methods are often made to improve the MRI image quality. MRI has excellent resolution and contrast among the soft tissues and displays good anatomical detail.

Nuclear medicine is the joining of nuclear physics, nuclear chemistry, and radiation detection. A radioactive chemical substance called a radiopharmaceutical is injected, usually intravenously (IV), where it concentrates in a particular tissue or organ of interest. The substance emits gamma rays that are detected by gamma cameras and then the captured gamma particles are counted by the camera. There are two principal gamma cameras: PET (positron emission tomography) and SPECT (single photon emission computed tomography). Nuclear imaging is often used to view physiological processes. For example, FDG-PET (florodeoxyglucose-PET) is frequently used to measure glucose metabolism, where the radiopharmaceutical (18) F-florodeoxyglucose is absorbed by every cell in the body. The higher the observed radioactivity as measured by PET, the higher the glucose metabolism. In some cancer studies, the malignant lesion has an increased glucose metabolism compared to the adjacent nonmalignant tissue and, thus, is useful in the diagnosis and staging of disease.

Another area where nuclear medicine is useful is in cardiac perfusion studies. For example, radiation therapy of esophageal cancer often induces

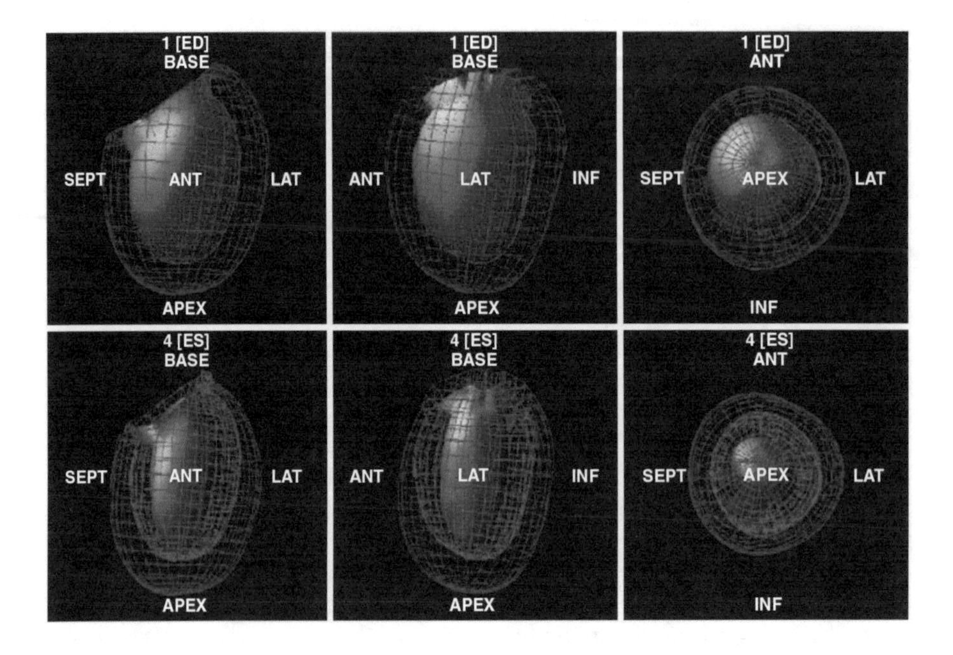

FIGURE 2.1
SPECT images of myocardial perfusion.

damage to the heart in the form of ischemia and scaring. The damage can be assessed by a nuclear medicine procedure, such as the exercise stress test, where thallium is administered via IV to the patient and concentrates in the heart muscle, and the resulting radioactivity is counted by SPECT to produce the image. Among the soft tissues, nuclear medicine procedures have fair-to-good contrast, but poor resolution and noise can be a problem for image quality. Figure 2.1 shows six SPECT images taken during one cycle of the heart for a myocardial perfusion study of Gayed[5] in order to determine the status of the heart of a cancer patient.

Ultrasonography (US) is the last modality to be described. It is based on a physical stream of energy passing through the body. The source is a transducer that converts electrical energy into a brief pulse of high-frequency acoustical energy to be transmitted into patient tissues. The transducer acts as a transmitter and receiver. The receiver detects echoes of sound deflected from the tissues, where the depth of a particular echo is measured by the round trip time of the transmitted emission. The images are viewed in real time on a monitor and the images are produced by interrogating patient tissue in the field of view. The real-time images are produced rapidly on the monitor allowing one to view moving tissue, such as respiration and cardiac motion. The US examination consists of applying the US transducer to the patient's skin using a water-soluble gel to make the connection secure for good transmission of the signal. Image quality is adversely affected by bone and by gas-filled structures, such as bowel and lung. For example, bone causes almost compete absorption of the signal producing an acoustic shadow on the image that hides the detail of tissues near the bone, while soft tissue, gas-filled objects produce a complete reflection of sound energy that eliminates visualization of deep structures. In spite of these drawbacks, the mode has many advantages, one of which is the noninvasive nature of the procedure. US is used to image a multitude of clinical challenges and is very beneficial when solving a particular clinical problem, such as viewing the development of a fetus.

Various modalities are often combined to improve overall diagnostic accuracy. For example, recently PET and CT have been combined to diagnose and stage esophageal cancer. When two modalities are combined, one must devise certain rules to decide when the combined procedure will produce a "positive" or "negative" determination. In another interesting study, US and CT were combined and their accuracy compared to FDG-PET. The ideas involved in measuring the accuracy of combined modalities will be outlined in Chapter 6.

It is important to remember, that the imaging device does not make the diagnosis, but rather the radiologist and others make the diagnosis. The modality is an aid to the radiologists and to others who are responsible for the treatment of the patient. After the radiologist reads the image, how is this information transformed to a scale where the biostatistician and others are able to use it for their own purposes?

For a nontechnical introduction to diagnostic imaging, Wolbarst[6] presents a very readable account. In addition, Jawad,[7] Chandra,[8] Seeram,[9] and Markisz and Aquilia[10] are standard references to cardiac ultrasound, nuclear medicine, computed tomography, and magnetic resonance imaging respectively.

2.3 Activities in Diagnostic Imaging

As stated earlier, diagnostic methods are ubiquitous in the healthcare system. These activities will be divided generally into two categories: (1) screening for preclinical disease, such as for breast cancer, heart disease, and lung cancer; and (2) as part of patient management during his/her stay in a large, modern healthcare facility. The emphasis in this book will be on the latter, where the patient has been diagnosed with the help of imaging and then is followed and monitored during his/her stay in the hospital. During the patient's stay, the following imaging activities are usually involved:

- Primary diagnosis or confirmation of earlier diagnoses.
- Diagnostic imaging to determine the extent of disease, including biopsy procedures, so-called staging studies, and follow-up medical procedures, such as surgery for biopsy or other forms of therapy.
- Monitoring the progression of the disease during therapy, such as in Phase II clinical trials.

Screening for disease, such as breast cancer, is performed to detect disease in the early phase, before symptoms appear. The early detection of disease when treatment is more effective and less expensive is the main objective of screening. It is assumed that early detection will lead to a more favorable diagnosis and that early treatment will be more effective than treatment given after symptoms appear. Another important goal of screening is to identify risk factors that would predispose the subject to a higher than average risk of developing disease. Imaging is almost always involved in the diagnosis of disease, but mammography is the only examination in wide use today as a screening tool. There are some other areas where screening is being tested, namely, in lung cancer with multidetector CT and in the detection of colorectal adenomatous polyps. One of the most important and difficult problems in clinical medicine is making recommendations for imaging studies for disease screening.

Screening should only be performed if the disease is serious and in the preclinical phase, and on a population that is at relatively high risk for developing the disease. Screening would not be effective if the disease can be effectively treated after the appearance of symptoms. If a false positive occurs, the patient is subjected to unnecessary follow-up procedures, such as surgery, additional imaging, and pathological testing for extent of the disease.

A diagnostic test, such as mammography, is efficacious only if it is accurate, that is, has good diagnostic characteristics, such as high sensitivity, specificity, and positive predictive value, and where a survival advantage can be demonstrated. How should a study be designed in order to evaluate the effectiveness of an imaging screening procedure? Of course, randomized studies have an advantage and are the basis for a recent article by Shen et al.[11] who reported on the survival advantage of screening detected cases over control groups. This investigation used data from three randomized studies with a total of 65,170 patients, and used Cox regression techniques to control for the so-called lead-time bias (detection of early stage disease with screening), tumor size, stage of disease, lymph node status, and age. They conclude that mammography screening is indeed effective. For additional information on the advantages of mammography, see Berry et al.[12] For recent Bayesian contributions to the estimation of sensitivity and lead-time in mammography, see Wu, Rosner, and Broemeling.[13,14]

The entire area of diagnostic screening has voluminous literature. This book will not focus on screening, and the reader is referred to Shen et al. who cite the most relevant studies. Some aspects of the Bayesian approach to screening for breast cancer is found in Chapter 9.

2.4 Accuracy and Agreement

How good is a diagnostic procedure? For example, suppose one is using mammography to diagnose breast cancer. How well does it correctly classify patients who have the disease and those who do not? Among those patients who have been classified with disease, what proportion actually has it? And, among those who were designated without disease, how many actually do not have it? To answer these questions, one must have a gold standard by which the true status of disease is determined. Thus, the gold standard will divide the patients into two groups: those with and those without the disease.

Another question is how does the radiologist decide when to classify an image as showing a malignant lesion? Often a confidence level scale is used where (1) designates definitely no malignancy, (2) probably no malignancy, (3) indeterminate, (4) probably a malignant lesion, and (5) definitely a malignant lesion. Given this diagnostic ordinal scale, how does the reader decide when to designate a patient as diseased? In the case of mammography, a score of 4 or 5 is often used to classify a patient as having the disease, in which case, each image can be classified as either (1) a true positive, (2) a true negative, (3) a false positive, and (4) a false negative. Of course, these four possibilities can only be used if one knows the true status of disease as given by the gold standard. Given these four outcomes, one may estimate the accuracy of the procedure with the usual measures of sensitivity, specificity, and positive and negative predictive values. For example, the specificity is estimated as the proportion of patients who test negative, among those who do not have the disease. There are many statistical methods to estimate test accuracy and will be explained in detail in Chapter 4. The idea of the area under the ROC curve will be explained and many examples introduced that will demonstrate its use as an overall measure of test accuracy.

Other factors that need to be taken into account are:

1. Design of the study.
2. Gold standard and how it is utilized.
3. Variability among and between observers and the input of others involved in diagnostic decisions.

With regard to the design, several questions must be asked. For example, how are the patients selected? Is one group of patients selected at random from a particular population or are two groups of patients, diseased and nondiseased, selected? Or, are they selected from patient charts, such as in a retrospective review? Along with this, what is the nature of the population from which the patients are selected? Is it a screening population, a community clinic, or a group of patients undergoing biopsies? These factors all affect the final determination of the accuracy as well as what biases will be introduced.

The gold standard often depends on surgery for biopsy, the pathology report from the lab, and additional imaging procedures. When and how the gold standard is used, often depends on the results of the diagnostic test. Often, only those who test positive for disease are subjected to the gold standard, while those who test negative are not. For example, with mammography, those who test positive are tested further with biopsy and tests for histology. While among those who test negative, follow-up of patient status is the gold standard.

Lastly, with regard to reader variability, it is important to remember that the diagnostic device is an aid to the people who make the diagnosis and that the diagnosis is made by group consensus (e.g., cardiologists, oncologists, surgeons, radiologists, pathologists, etc.). All of this introduces variability and error into the final determination of disease status.

Is agreement between and among observers (radiologists, pathologists, surgeons, etc.) an important component of diagnostic medicine? Of course it is. Suppose a Phase II clinical trial is being conducted to determine the efficacy of new treatment for advanced prostate cancer with, say, 35 patients. The major endpoint is tumor response to therapy, which is based on the change in tumor size from baseline to some future time point. Often the percent change from baseline is used and, furthermore, this determination depends on the readings of the same images of several radiologists. Since they differ in regard to training and experience, their determination of the change varies from reader to reader. How is this taken into account? How is a consensus reached?

Statistical methods that consider and measure agreement are well developed. For example, with ordinal test scores, agreement between observers is often measured by the Kappa statistic, while, if the test score is continuous, regression techniques for calibration (e.g., Bland-Altman) are frequently ordered to assess accuracy within and between observers. Analysis of variance techniques that account for various sources (patients, readers, modalities, replications, etc.) of variability help in estimating the between and within reader variability via the intra-class correlation coefficient. In Chapter 4 and Chapter 5, test accuracy and agreement between observers will be revealed in detail.

Kundel and Polansky[15] give a brief introduction to the various issues concerning the measurement of agreement between observers in diagnostic imaging, and Shoukri[16] has an excellent book on the subject.

2.5 Developmental Trials for Imaging

When developing a new imaging modality, the diagnostic procedure must successfully complete three phases labeled I, II, and III. This is similar to the designation for patient clinical trials, but what is referred to here is for the development of medical devices. The different phases are for different objectives of test accuracy.

Phase I consists of exploratory trials and is usually retrospective with 10 to 50 patients and 2 to 3 readers. There are two populations, a homogenous group of diseased subjects who are definitely known to have the disease, and a second group of homogenous people definitely known not to have the disease. The key word here is homogenous, where the symptoms of the disease are more or less the same among diseased patients, while the nondiseased are healthy in the same way. The accuracy is measured by true positive and false positive rates as well as the area under the ROC curve. Thus, if the accuracy is not good, the modality needs to be improved. (See Bogaert et al.[17] for a good example of Phase I developmental trial involving MRI angiography.)

If a device has sufficient accuracy during Phase I, it is then studied in Phase II trials. These trials, also called challenge trials, typically enroll 50 to 200 cases and 5 to 10 observers. Like Phase I trials, Phase II trials are also retrospective, but with a wide spectrum of the disease in the two groups. Thus, if the disease is nonsmall cell lung cancer, patients with different manifestations (different ages, different stages of disease, and patients who have disease similar to nonsmall cell lung cancer) of disease are included. It is more difficult for the device to distinguish between diseased and nondiseased subjects. Among the nondiseased, the patients are also heterogeneous. Test accuracy is measured as in a Phase I trial, and the association between accuracy and the pathological, clinical, and co-morbid features of the patient can be investigated with regression modeling. The comparison between digital radiography and conventional chest imaging was performed as a Phase II trial by Theate et al.[18]

Beam et al.[19] investigated the interpretation of screening mammograms as a Phase III trial using 108 readers, 79 images read twice by each reader, and many healthcare centers. The sensitivity (proportion of patients among the diseased who test positive) ranged from .47 to 1 and specificity (proportion of patients who do not have the disease who test negative) from .36 to .99 across readers. Phase III trials are prospective and are designed to estimate test performance in a well-defined clinical population and involve at least 10 observers, several hundred cases, and competing modalities. A device should pass all three phases before becoming a standard in a general clinical setting.

Note that it is important to know the inter-observer variability in these trials because the accuracy of the modality depends not only on the device, but the interpretation of the image via the various readers. Pepe gives more detail, in Chapter 8, in the description of developmental trials, and Obuchowski[21] provides sample size tables for the number of observers and the number of patients in trials for device development.

2.6 Protocol Review and Clinical Trials

As we have seen, diagnostic procedures are performed in all areas of patient care, and now we will see just how it appears in the patient's experience with clinical trials. First, we examine the essential elements of a protocol, the protocol review process, and the role diagnostic imaging in Phase II trials. Crowley's[22] book is an excellent reference to statistical consideration in clinical trials.

2.6.1 The Protocol

Protocol states in detail how the medical study is organized and executed. There are several types: cooperative group protocols, National Cancer Institute (NCI) protocols, those submitted by a pharmaceutical or medical device company, and those that are initiated by a principal investigator at the institution. The protocol should include the following components:

1. An explanation of the scientific basis for the study.
2. A summary of the results of all previous related studies and experiments of the study intervention.
3. Patient eligibility and ineligibility criteria.
4. A list of the major and minor endpoints, including their definitions and how and when they will be measured.
5. Definitions of evaluable and intent-to-treat populations.
6. Estimated patient accrual rates by site.
7. A statistical section that outlines a detailed power analysis for sample size, a description of rules for stopping early, methods for randomizing patients, and the proposed statistical analysis.
8. Nonstatistical stopping rules for safety considerations.

Additional documentation that must accompany the protocol is a list of all NCI toxicities and the patient-informed consent form. For protocols initiated by private companies, a biostatistician is assigned to review it, but for protocols initiated at MDACC, the study has one biostatistician assigned as a collaborator (the one who assisted the principal investigator (PI) in the statistical design) and a different statistician who reviews the protocol and presents it to the department for approval.

Every protocol at MDACC is reviewed in three steps: first by the Department of Biostatistics and Applied Mathematics, then by the Clinical Research Committee (CRC), and lastly by the Institutional Review Board (IRB). During the first review, a biostatistician presents the protocol in written and oral form to the department, where there is a set procedure for this presentation. The presentation is concluded with a list of major and minor concerns regarding the revision of the protocol. The department then discusses the above-mentioned tentative revisions and votes to approve a directive to be sent to the PI. If need be, the PI then revises the protocol accordingly, often with the help of the biostatistical collaborator and/or the reviewer.

2.6.2 Phase I, II, and III Clinical Designs

The important role played by diagnostic imaging in clinical trials can be found in Chapter 8, and the following briefly describes Phase I, II, and III clinical trials. Phase I trials evaluate how a treatment is to be administered and how that treatment affects the human body. First, consider a Phase I study that evaluates safety among a set of doses of a new treatment. The study will be designed to determine the maximum tolerable dose (MTD), which is the dose whereby at higher doses the safety of the patient would be compromised. One is assuming that as the dose level increases, the probability of toxicity increases and the probability of efficacy also increases. The main endpoint in a Phase I study is a measure of toxicity experienced by the patient as a result of the treatment, while the secondary endpoint is a measure of efficacy. To define the toxicity endpoint, the investigator characterizes the dose limiting toxicity (DLT), which is a set of toxicities that are severe enough to prevent giving more of the treatment at higher doses. The investigator bases the DLT on knowledge of the disease, treatment, and the patients who are eligible for the trial. Investigators are guided by the NCI list of common toxicities or in some other manner that is appropriate for the particular study. Phase I trial objectives may include the study of the pharmacokinetics and pharmacodynamics of the drug; however, we will not emphasize this here. Primarily, the goal of Phase I studies is to profile the toxicity of the drug or intervention using a set of doses and a well-defined DLT.

Once a particular treatment or intervention has been studied with a Phase I trial and the MTD has been selected and we are satisfied that the treatment will be safe, studies of the treatment may progress to Phase II trials to determine if the treatment holds sufficient promise. Typically, the target population is patients with a specific disease, disease site, histology, or stage, or patients undergoing some surgical or anesthetic procedure. Often the treatment dose is the MTD determined from previous Phase I trials. Although limited dose finding is sometimes allowed to accommodate different patient populations, the primary endpoints are measures of efficacy, while safety is secondary.

Diagnostic imaging plays a crucial role in Phase II trials. Often the primary endpoint is the fraction of patients who experience a response to therapy, and often the response is based on the change in tumor size as measured from baseline to some future point at the end of the treatment cycle. Thus, the major endpoint in such a study is a diagnostic one provided by radiologists.

We are now at the point where we have an intervention (drug or procedure) that has been studied in a series of Phase I and Phase II trials and has demonstrated sufficient promise to be compared to the standard clinical treatment in a large randomized study.

Phase III trials are confirmatory, where the study procedure is to be compared to the standard therapy with the goal of providing evidence that the study drug will provide substantial improvement in survival time, in disease-free survival, or some other time-to-event endpoint, such as time to response or time to hospitalization, etc. They should be designed to have a sufficient sample size to detect clinically relevant differences and are usually done in a multicenter setting. Provisions are made for an interim look by an independent Data Safety Monitoring Board (DSMB), where the trial may be stopped early for reasons of safety and/or efficacy.

2.7 The Literature

As mentioned earlier, biostatistics play a pivotal role in the imaging literature, as can be discerned by reading articles in the mainline journals, such as *Academic Radiology, The American Journal of Roentgenology,* and *Radiology,* and the more specialized, such as *The Journal of Computed Assisted Tomography, The Journal of Magnetic Resonance Imaging, The Journal of Nuclear Medicine,* and *Ultrasound in Medicine.*

For some reference books in the area of general diagnostic imaging, the standard one is *Fundamentals of Diagnostic Radiology,* edited by Brant and Helms.[23] This book is primarily for radiologists and discusses the fundamentals of imaging principals and provides a description of the latest clinical applications.

Two relevant statistical books are *The Statistical Evaluation of Medical Tests for Classification and Prediction* by Pepe[20] and *Statistical Methods in Diagnostic Medicine* by Zhou, McClish, and Obuchowski.[24] Both are excellent and intended for biostatisticians.

References

1. Mielke, C.H., Shields, J.P., and Broemeling, L.D., Coronary artery calcium scores for men and women of a large asymptomatic population, *Cardiovasc. Dis. Preven.,* 2, 194, 1992.
2. Mielke, C.H., Shields J.P., and Broemeling, L.D., Coronary artery calcium, coronary artery disease, and diabetes. *Diabetes Res. Clin. Pract.,* 53, 55, 2001.
3. Mielke, C.H., Shields, J.P., and Broemeling, L.D., Risk factors and coronary artery disease for asymptomatic women using electron beam computed tomography. *J. Cardiol. Risk,* 8, 81, 2001.
4. Dasgupta, N., Xie, P., Cheney, M.O., Broemeling, L., and Mielke, C.H., The Spokane heart study: Weibull regression and coronary artery disease, *Commun. Stat. Simul.,* 29, 747, 2000.
5. Gayed, I., Personal Communication, Department of Diagnostic Imaging, The University of Texas MD Anderson Cancer Center, 2006.
6. Wolbarst, A.B., *Looking within: How X-ray, CT, MRI, and Ultrasound and Other Medical Images Are Created and How They Help Physicians Save Lives,* University of California Press, 1999, Berkeley.
7. Jawad, I.J., *A Practical Guide to Echocardiography and Cardiac Doppler Ultrasound* (2nd ed.), Little Brown and Company, 1996, Boston.
8. Chandra, R., *Nuclear Medicine Physics, the Basics,* Williams and Wilkins, 1998, Baltimore.
9. Seeram, E., *Computed Tomography, Clinical Applications, and Quality Control,* (2nd ed.), W.B. Saunders Company, 2001, Philadelphia.
10. Markisz, J.A. and Aguilia, M., *Technical Magnetic Imaging,* Appleton and Lange, 1996, Stamford, CT.

11. Shen, Y., Inoue, L.Y.T., Munsell, M.F., Miller, A.B., and Berry, D.A., Role of detection method in predicting breast cancer survival: analysis of randomized screening trials, *J. Nat. Cancer Inst.*, 97, 1195, 2005.
12. Berry, D.A. et al., Effect of screening and adjuvant therapy on mortality from breast cancer, *N. Engl. J. Med.*, 353(17), 1784, 2005.
13. Wu, D., Rosner G., and Broemeling, L.D., MLE and Bayesian inferences of age-dependent sensitivity and transition probability in periodic screening, *Biometrics*, 61, 1056, 2005.
14. Wu, D., Rosner, G., and Broemeling, L.D., Bayesian inference for the lead time in periodic cancer screening, (in press) *Biometrics* 2006.
15. Kundel, H.L. and Polansky, M., Measure of observer agreement, *Radiology*, 228, 303, 2003.
16. Shoukri, M.M., *Measures of Interobserver Agreement*, Chapman & Hall/ CRC, 2002, Boca Raton, FL.
17. Bogaert, J., Kuzo, R., Dymarkowski, S., Becker, R., Piessens, J., and Rademaker, F.E., Coronary artery imaging with real-time navigator three dimensional turbo field echo MR coronary angiography: initial experience, *Radiology*, 226, 707, 2003.
18. Theate, F.L., Fuhrman, C.R., Oliver, J.H., et al., Digital radiography and conventional imaging of the chest: a comparison of observer performance, *Am. J. Roentgeneol.*, 162, 575,1994.
19. Beam, C.A., Lyde, P.M., and Sullivan, D.C., Variability in the interpretation of screening mammograms by U.S. radiologists, *Arch. Int. Med.*, 156, 209,1996.
20. Pepe, M.S., *The Statistical Evaluation of Medical Tests for Classification and Prediction*, Oxford University Press, 2003, Oxford, U.K.
21. Obuchowski, N.A. Sample size tables for receiver operating characteristic studies, *Am. J. Roentgenol.*, 175, 603, 2000.
22. Crowley, J., *Handbook of Statistics in Clinical Oncology*, Marcel Dekker, 2001, New York.
23. Brant, W.E. and Helms, C.A., *Fundamentals of Diagnostic Imaging*, (2nd ed.), Lippincott, Williams, and Wilkins, 1999, New York.
24. Zhou, H.H., McClish, D.K., and Obuchowski, N.A., *Statistical Methods for Diagnostic Medicine*, John Wiley & Sons, 2002, New York.

Chapter 3

Other Diagnostic Procedures

3.1 Introduction

Several stages are involved in the determination of a definitive diagnosis. For example, a screening mammography might reveal a suspicious lesion, which is followed with a biopsy of the lesion. Also, many people are involved in the diagnostic process and, as has been emphasized, diagnostic imaging plays a major role in that effort. In addition to radiologists, there are oncologists, surgeons, nurses, pathologists, and geneticists. The pathologists play a crucial role in performing the histologic tests on cell specimens taken from a biopsy, as does the microbiologist and geneticist, who are developing new techniques that measure gene sensitivity from DNA specimens. Three examples are described below: (1) diagnosis of metastasis of the primary melanoma lesion to the lymph nodes, (2) a biopsy of lung nodules, and (3) screening for coronary artery disease with CT.

3.2 Sentinel Lymph Node Biopsy for Melanoma

The sentinel lymph node (SLN) biopsy is employed to diagnose the metastasis of many forms of cancer including breast, prostate, and lung. Its use in melanoma is outlined below.

The technique involves the cooperation of a melanoma oncologist, a surgical team to dissect the lymph nodes, diagnostic radiologists who will perform the nuclear medicine procedure, and pathologists who examine the lymph node samples. The following description of the technique is based on Pawlik and Gershenwald.[1] The early procedures are described by Morton et al.[2] and consisted of injecting a blue dye intradermally around the primary lesion and biopsy site where the lymphatic system takes up the dye and carries it, via afferent lymphatics, to the draining regional node basins. Surgeons then explore the draining nodal basin and the first draining lymph nodes. The SLNs are identified by their uptake of blue dye, dissected and sent to pathology for histological examination of malignancy.

These early methods were recently revised to include a nuclear medicine application using a handheld gamma camera. (See Gershenwald et al.[3] for a good explanation of this.) With this technique, intra-operative mapping uses a handheld gamma probe, where .5 to 1.0 mCi (millicurie) of a radiopharmaceutical is injected intradermally around the intact melanoma. The gamma camera monitors the level of radioactivity from the injection sites to the location of the SLNs and is also employed to assist the surgeons with the dissection of the lymph nodes. This probe is used transcutaneously prior to surgery and has an accuracy of 96 to 99% in the correct identification of the SLNs. Histological examination of the lymph node specimens determine if the lymph node basin has malignant melanoma cells.

3.3 Tumor Depth to Diagnose Metastatic Melanoma

A SLN biopsy for melanoma metastasis is illustrated in a recent study by Rousseau et al.[4] where the records of 1376 melanoma patients were reviewed. The main objective was to diagnose metastasis to the lymph nodes where the gold standard is the outcome of the SLN biopsy and the diagnosis is made on the basis of tumor depth of the primary lesion, the Clark level of the primary, the age and gender of the patient, the presence of an ulcerated primary, and the site (axial or extremity) of the primary lesion. The overall incidence of a positive biopsy was 16.9%, the median age was 51 years, and 58% were male. A multivariate analysis with logistic regression showed that tumor thickness and ulceration were highly significant in predicting SLN status. For additional details about this study, refer to Rousseau et al., but here the focus will be on tumor thickness for the diagnosis of lymph node metastasis.

How accurate is tumor thickness for the diagnosis of lymph node metastasis? The original measurement of tumor thickness was categorized into four groups: (1) ≤1 mm, (2) 1.01 to 2.00 mm, (3) 2.01 to 4.00 mm, and (4) > 4.00 mm. If groups 3 and 4 are used to designate a positive (lymph node metastasis) test and groups 1 and 2 a negative test, the sensitivity and specificity are calculated as 156/234 = .666 and 832/1147 = .725, respectively. There were 234 patients with a positive SLN biopsy and, among those, 156 had a tumor thickness greater than 2.00 mm; on the other hand, there were 832 patients with a tumor thickness of ≤2.00 mm among 1147 with a negative SLN biopsy. Also, using the original continuous measurement and a conventional estimation method, the area under the receiving operating characteristic (ROC) curve is .767 with a standard deviation of .016.

This type of problem will be studied in the chapters to come, but from a Bayesian perspective.

3.4 Biopsy for Nonsmall Cell Lung Cancer

At the MD Anderson Cancer Center (MDACC), the Department of Interventional Radiology is part of the Division of Diagnostic Imaging and where they perform invasive biopsy procedures. For example, they perform biopsies of lung lesions using a computed tomography (CT)-guided technique (see Gupta et al.[5]). The Gupta example described below compares two methods of biopsy, short vs. long needle path, for target lesions less than 2 cm in size. The objective is to retrieve a specimen of the lesion to be examined for malignancy by a cytopathologist.

Many people are involved, including those assisting the interventional radiologist in guiding the needle to the target lesion, which was earlier detected and located by various imaging modalities. Of main concern is the occurrence of a pneumothorax, which can result in a collapsed lung and bleeding, sometimes requiring a chest tube for draining fluid from the chest cavity.

This cohort study included 176 patients (79 men and 97 women, ranging in age from 18 to 84 years). This was not a randomized study, and patient information came from all persons who underwent a CT-guided biopsy for lung nodules during the period from November 1, 2000 to December 31, 2002. There were two groups: Group A with 48 patients, where the needle path was less than 1 cm in length of aerated lung, and Group B with 128 patients, where the needle path length was greater than 1 cm.

The two groups were similar with regard to age, gender, lesion size, and lesion location. The major endpoints were diagnostic yield (number of diagnostic samples and test accuracy, measured by sensitivity and specificity) and frequency of pneumothorax. The report from pathology served as a gold standard for test accuracy.

The statistical analysis consisted of estimating test accuracy of the two methods and comparing accuracy via the chi-square test. There was no significant difference between the two groups with regard to sensitivity and specificity; however there were significant differences between the two with regard to complications from the procedure. For example, the pneumothorax rate of $35/48 = .73$ was larger for the short needle path group compared to $38/128 = .29$ for the long needle path group.

As a follow-up to this, a recent study of 191 lung biopsy patients who experienced pneumothorax, was performed. In that study, the principal aim was to identify those factors that significantly impact the development of a persistent air leak of the lung.

3.5 Coronary Artery Disease

A common scenario in the diagnosis of coronary artery disease is as follows. Following complaints of chest pain, the patient undergoes an exercise stress test and, if necessary, followed by an angiogram, a catheterization of the coronary arteries. There are several experimental studies that involve a CT determination of the coronary artery calcium (CAC) in the coronary arteries. One such study involved 1958 men and 1281 women who were referred to the Shields Coronary Artery Center in Spokane, WA over the period from January 1990 to May 1998. Some of the subjects had been diagnosed with coronary artery disease, while others were referred because they were suspected of having the disease. Measurements of CAC were made with the GE Imatron C-100 Ultrafast CT Scanner. (See Mielke et al.[6] for more details of the Spokane study.) In Chapter 5 of this book, the diagnostic accuracy of CAC is examined with a Bayesian technique for this study.

Another way to diagnose coronary artery disease is to measure the degree of stenosis in the arteries by magnetic resonance angiography. For example, Obuchowski[7] used the results of a study by Masaryk et al.[8] to illustrate a nonparametric way of estimating the area under the ROC curve for clustered data. There were two readers and two measurements per patient, one for the left and one for the right coronary arteries, and the correlation introduced by this clustering effect was taken into account by Obuchowski's analysis. This makes a perfect example for comparing readers, and a Bayesian analog is introduced in Chapter 5.

References

1. Pawlik, T.M., and Gershenwald, J.E., Sentinel lymph node biopsy for melanoma, *Contemp. Surg.*, 61(4), 175, 2005.
2. Morton, D.L., Wanek, L., Nizze, J.A., Elashoff, R.M., and Wong, J.H., Improved long term survival lymphadenectomy of melanoma metastatic to regional lymph nodes: analysis of prognostic factors in 1134 patients from the John Wayne Cancer Center Institute, *Ann. Surg.*, 214, 491,1991.
3. Gershenwald, J.E., Tseng, C.H., Thompson, W., et al., Improved sentinel lymph node localization in patients with primary melanoma with the use of radio labeled colloid, *Surgery*, 124, 203,1998.
4. Rousseau, D.L., Ross, M.I., Johnson, M.M., Prieto, V.G., Lee, J.E., Mansfield, P.F., and Gershenwald, J.E., Revised American Joint Committee on Cancer Staging Criteria accurately predict sentinel lymph node positivity in clinically node negative melanoma patients, *Ann. Surg. Oncol.*, 10(5), 569, 2003.
5. Gupta, S., Krishnamurthy, S., Broemeling, L.D., Morello, F.A., Wallace, M.J., Ahrar, K., Madoff, D.L., Murthy, R., and Hicks, M.E., Small (<2 cm) sub pleural pulmonary lesions; short versus long needle path, CT-guided biopsy: comparison of diagnostic yields and complications, *Radiology*, 234, 631, 2005.

6. Mielke, H.C., Shields, P.J., and Broemeling, L.D., Coronary artery calcium scores for men and women of a large asymptomatic population, *Cardiovas. Dis. Preven.*, 2, 194, 1999.
7. Obuchowski, N.A., Non parametric analysis of clustered ROC curve data, *Biometrics*, 53, 567, 1997.
8. Masaryk, A.M., Ross, J.S., DiCello, M.C., Modic, M.T., Paranandi, L., and Masaryk, T.J., Angiography of the carotid bifurcation: potential and limitations as a screening examination, *Radiology*, 121, 337, 1991.

Chapter 4

Bayesian Statistics

4.1 Introduction

The previous three chapters presented the scientific background necessary in order to appreciate the statistical applications that will be encountered in Chapter 4 through Chapter 9. Bayesian methods will be employed to design and analyze studies in medical diagnostics. This chapter describes Bayesian inference by introducing Bayes theorem, the foundation of the subject. This is followed with a description of the theorem: The prior information from the sample given by the likelihood function and the posterior distribution, which is the basis of all inferential techniques in Bayesian statistics. Next is a description of the main two elements of inference, namely estimation and tests of hypotheses. Also included is a demonstration of the Bayesian predictive density, another important component of inference.

The remaining sections of the chapter list the important distributions for Bayesian inference, including the binomial, Beta, multinomial, Dirichlet, normal, gamma, normal-gamma, and the univariate and multivariate t-distributions. These are used to analyze the accuracy of diagnostic tests. Next, the previous distributions are illustrated by making Bayesian inferences for diagnostic accuracy in imaging studies: a Bayesian principle.

Of course, inferential procedures can only be applied if there is adequate computing available. If the posterior distribution is known, analytical methods are often sufficient to implement Bayesian inferences, or direct sampling from the posterior distribution will give the necessary information. Direct sampling is easily done if the relevant random number generators are available. On the other hand, if the posterior distribution is quite complicated and not a recognized standard distribution and/or random number generators are not available, it is often necessary to generate samples from the posterior distribution by indirect means. To address this problem, Monte Carlo Markov Chain (MCMC) techniques have been developed over the past 25 years and have been a major contributor to the successful application of Bayesian methods for the analysis of complicated problems.

Minitab®, S-plus®, SAS®, and other packages provide random number generators for direct sampling from the posterior distribution for many standard posterior distributions. For indirect sampling, WinBUGS® (which employs Gibbs sampling, the Metropolis-Hasting (MH) algorithm, and hybrid Gibbs/MH algorithms) is a good alternative. At the MD Anderson Cancer Center (MDACC), where Bayesian applications are routine, several special purpose programs are available for designing (including sample size justification) and analyzing clinical trials and will be described in a later section of this chapter.

4.2 Bayes Theorem

Suppose X is a continuous observable random vector and $\theta \in \Omega \subset R^m$ is an unknown parameter vector, and suppose the conditional density of X given θ is denoted by $f(x/\theta)$, then the conditional density of θ, given $X = x$, is

$$\xi(\theta/x) = c\ f(x/\theta)\ \xi(\theta), \quad \theta \in \Omega \quad \text{and} \quad x \in R. \tag{4.1}$$

The normalizing constant $c > 0$ is chosen so that the integral of $f(x/\theta)\ \xi(\theta)$ with respect to θ is unity. The above equation is referred to as Bayes theorem and is the foundation of all statistical inferences to be employed in the analysis of data. If X is discrete, $f(x/\theta)$ is the probability mass function of X. The density $\xi(\theta)$ is the prior density of θ and represents the knowledge one possesses about the parameter before one observes X. This prior information is most likely available to the experimenter from other previous related experiments. Note that θ is considered a random variable and that Bayes theorem transforms one's prior knowledge of θ, represented by its prior density, to the posterior density, and that the transformation is the combining of the prior information about θ with the sample information represented by $f(x/\theta)$. If $x = (x_1, x_2, \ldots, x_n)$ represents a random sample of size n from the sample space, then Bayes theorem is given by

$$\xi(\theta/x) \propto \prod_{i=1}^{i=n} f(x_i/\theta)\ \xi(\theta), \quad x_i \in R \quad \text{and} \quad \in \Omega \tag{4.2}$$

where the proportionality is with respect to θ. The term $\prod_{i=1}^{i=n} f(x_i/\theta)$ is called the likelihood function of θ and is the information one has about θ as induced by the sample information.

The beginnings of our subject is "an essay toward solving a problem in the doctrine of chances" by the Rev. Thomas Bayes.[1] He considered a binomial experiment with n trials and assumed the probability θ of success was uniformly distributed and presented a way to calculate $Pr(a \le \theta \le b / X = p)$, where X is the number of successes in n independent trials. This was a first in the sense that Bayes was making inferences via $\xi(\theta/x)$, the conditional density of θ, given $X = x$. Also, by assuming the parameter was uniformly distributed, he was assuming vague prior information for θ.

Arguably, Laplace[2,3] made the greatest contributions to inverse probability (he was unaware of Bayes) beginning in 1774 with "Memorie sur la probabilite des causes par la evenemens," with his own version of Bayes theorem. His contributions spanned a period of some 40 years and culminated in "Theorie analytique des probabilites." (See Stigler[4] and Chapter 9 through Chapter 20 of Hald[5,6] for the history of Laplace's monumental contributions to inverse probability.)

It was in relatively modern times that Bayesian statistics began its resurgence with works by Lhoste,[7] Jeffreys,[8] Savage,[9] and Lindley.[10] According to Broemeling and Broemeling,[11] Lhoste was the first to justify noninformative priors by invariance principals, a tradition carried on by Jeffreys. Savage's book was a major contribution in that Bayesian inference and decision theory were put on a sound theoretical footing as a consequence of certain axioms of probability and utility. Lindley's two volumes illustrated the relevance of Bayesian inference to everyday statistical problems and was quite influential and set the tone and style for later books, such as Box and Tiao,[12] Zellner,[13] and Broemeling.[14] Box and Tiao and Broemeling presented Bayesian methods for the usual statistical problems of the analysis of variance and regression, while Zellner focused Bayesian methods on certain regression problems in econometrics. During this period, inferential problems were solved analytically or by numerical integration. Models with many parameters (such as hierarchical models with many levels) were difficult to use because, at that time, numerical integration methods had limited capability in higher dimensions. (For a good history of Bayesian (inverse probability) inference, see Chapter 3 of Stigler and the two volumes of Hald, which present a comprehensive history and are invaluable as a reference.)

The past 20 years is characterized by the development of resampling techniques where samples are generated from the posterior distribution via MCMC methods, such as Gibbs sampling. Because the computing technology is available, large samples generated from the posterior make it possible to make statistical inferences and to employ multilevel hierarchical models to solve complex but practical problems. (See Leonard and Hsu,[15] Gelman et al.,[16] Congdon,[17–19] Carlin and Louis,[20] who demonstrate the utility of MCMC techniques in Bayesian statistics.)

4.3 Prior Information

Bayesian inference is initiated with prior information, a crucial component of Bayes rule (Equation (4.2)). Bayes assumed the prior distribution of the parameter is uniform, namely

$$\xi(\theta) = 1, \quad 0 \le \theta \le 1, \tag{4.3}$$

where θ is probability of success in n independent trials and

$$f(x/\theta) = \binom{n}{x}\theta^x(1-\theta)^{n-x}, \tag{4.4}$$

where x is the number of successes $= 0, 1, 2, \ldots, n$. The conditional distribution of X, the number of successes is binomial and denoted by $X \sim \text{Binomial}(\theta, n)$. The uniform prior was used for many years, until Lhoste employed

$$\xi(\theta) = \theta^{-1}(1-\theta)^{-1}, \quad 0 \le \theta \le 1, \tag{4.5}$$

to represent prior information that is noninformative and an improper density function. Lhoste[7] based this prior on certain invariance principals, quite similar to what Jeffreys[8] did in 1931. Lhoste also developed a noninformative prior for the standard deviation σ of a normal population with density

$$f(x/\theta,\sigma) = \left(1/\sqrt{2\pi\sigma}\right)\exp-(1/2\sigma)(x-\mu)^2, \quad \mu \in R \quad \text{and} \quad \sigma > 0. \tag{4.6}$$

Lhoste used invariance as follows. He reasoned that the prior density of σ and the prior density of $1/\sigma$ should be the same, and this led to

$$\xi(\sigma) = 1/\sigma. \tag{4.7}$$

Jeffreys used the same approach in developing noninformative priors for binomial and normal populations, but also developed noninformative priors for multiparameter models, including the mean and standard deviation for the normal density as

$$\xi(\mu,\sigma) = 1/\sigma, \quad \mu \in R \quad \text{and} \quad \sigma > 0. \tag{4.8}$$

Noninformative priors where ubiquitous from the 1920s to the 1980s and were included in all the textbooks of that era. For example, see Box and Tiao,[12] Zellner,[13] and Broemeling.[14]

Looking back, it is somewhat ironic that noninformative priors were almost always used, even though informative prior information was almost always available. This limited the utility of the Bayesian approach, and people saw very little advantage over the conventional way of doing business. The major strength of the Bayesian way is that it a convenient, practical, and logical method of utilizing informative prior information. Surely, the investigator knows informative prior information from previous related studies.

How does one express informative information with a prior density? For example, suppose one has informative prior information for the binomial population (Equation (4.4)). Consider

$$\xi(\theta) = [\Gamma(\alpha+\beta)/\Gamma(\alpha)\Gamma(\beta)]\theta^{\alpha-1}(1-\theta)^{\beta-1}, \quad 0 \le \theta \le 1, \tag{4.9}$$

as the prior density for θ.

For example, suppose from a previous study with 20 trials, there were 6 successes and 14 failures, then the probability mass function for the observed number of successes $x = 6$ is

$$f(6/\theta) = \binom{20}{6} \theta^6(1-\theta)^{14}, \quad 0 \le \theta \le 1. \tag{4.10}$$

As a function of θ, Equation (4.10) is the likelihood function for θ, which is a Beta (7,15) density and expresses informative prior information, which will be combined with Equation (4.4), via Bayes theorem, in order to make inferences (estimation, tests of hypotheses, and predictions) about the parameter. The Beta distribution is an example of a conjugate density because the prior and posterior distributions for θ belong to the same parametric family. Thus, the likelihood function based on previous sample information can serve as a source of informative prior information. The binomial and Beta distributions occur quite frequently in diagnostic medicine, as, for example, in Phase II clinical trials and in estimating the accuracy of diagnostic tests.

Of course, the normal density (Equation (4.6)) also plays an important role as a population model in diagnostic imaging, when the diagnostic variable is a continuous measurement. How is informative prior information expressed for μ and σ? Suppose a previous study has m observations $x = (x_1, x_2, \ldots, x_m)$, then the density of x, given μ and σ, is

$$f(x/\mu,\sigma) \propto \left[\sqrt{m}/\sqrt{2\pi\sigma^2}\right] \exp-(m/2\sigma^2)(\bar{x}-\mu)^2$$

$$[(2\pi)^{-(n-1)/2}\sigma^{-(n-1)}] \exp-(1/2\sigma^2)\sum_{i-1}^{i=m}(x_i-\bar{x})^2. \tag{4.11}$$

This is a conjugate density for the two-parameter normal family and is called the normal-inverse gamma density. It is the product of two functions, where the first, as a function of μ and σ, is the conditional density of μ given σ with mean $\bar{x}$ and variance σ^2/m, while the second function is a function of σ only and is an inverse gamma.

Thus, if one knows the results of a previous experiment, the likelihood function for μ and τ provides informative prior information for the normal population. Such prior information will be relevant when considering estimation of the area under the receiving operating characteristic (ROC) curve for continuous diagnostic test data.

TABLE 4.1

Mortality Study: Deaths/Total

Trial	Treated	Control
1	3/38	3/39
2	7/114	14/116
3	5/69	11/93
4	102/1533	127/1520
...	...	...
20	32/209	40/218
21	27/391	43/364
22	22/680	39/674

With the advent of MCMC techniques for sampling the posterior distribution of complex hierarchical models, prior information is expressed in a more complex fashion because there are several levels of parameters. Such an example is taken from volume 1 of the help section of version 1.4 of WinBUGS and is based on a study by Carlin[21] who considered a Bayesian approach to meta-analysis, and includes the following example of 22 trials of beta blockers to prevent mortality after myocardial infarction (Table 4.1).

The following are the program statements:

```
model
{
for( i in 1 : Num ) {
rc[i] ~ dbin(pc[i], nc[i])
rt[i] ~ dbin(pt[i], nt[i])
logit(pc[i]) <- m[i]
logit(pt[i]) <- m[i] + d[i]                    (4.12)
m[i] ~ dnorm(0.0,1.0E-5)
d[i] ~ dnorm(delta, tau)
}
delta ~ dnorm(0.0,1.0E-6)
tau ~ dgamma(0.001,0.001)
delta.new ~ dnorm(d, tau)
sigma <- 1 / sqrt(tau)
}
```

For each trial, a different probability of a success is given for the control and treatment groups, and the probabilities are transformed to the logit scale, then the parameters of the logit are given normal noninformative priors. Thus, the *m*s are given independent normal distributions with mean 0.0 and precision .00001. The *d*s are given a normal (delta, tau) distribution, and the delta is given a normal (0.0, .000001) distribution. There are three levels of parameters involved in this example. The success probabilities, the logit parameters, namely the *ms* and *ds*, and finally at the third stage the normal (0.0, .000001) distribution for delta, which is the mean of the second level *d* parameters.

Another third level parameter is the precision tau of the delta parameters, which is given a noninformative gamma (0.001, .001) distribution. The tau parameter is the inverse of the variance. The main parameter of interest is delta because, if it is zero, there is no difference in mortality between the control and treatment groups. We will return to this example when discussing Gibbs sampling.

4.4 Posterior Information

The preceding section explained how prior information is expressed in an informative or vague way. Several examples were given and these will be revisited to determine the posterior distribution of the parameters.

In the Bayes example, where $X \sim$ Binomial (θ, n), a uniform distribution for θ was used. What is the posterior distribution? By Bayes theorem

$$\xi(\theta/x) \propto \binom{n}{x} \theta^{x}(1-\theta)^{n-x}, \tag{4.13}$$

where x is the observed number of successes in n trials. Of course, this is recognized as a Beta $(x + 1, n - x + 1)$ distribution with a posterior mean of $(x + 1)/(n + 2)$. On the other hand, if the Lhoste prior

$$\xi(\theta) = \theta^{-1}(1-\theta)^{-1}, \quad 0 \le \theta \le 1,$$

is used, the posterior distribution of θ is Beta $(x, n - x)$ with mean x/n, the usual estimator of θ. The conjugate prior (Equation (4.9)) results in a Beta $(x+\alpha, n-x+\beta)$ with mean $(x+\alpha)/(n+\alpha+\beta)$. Suppose the prior is informative with a previous 10 successes in 30 trials, then $\alpha = 11$ and $\beta = 21$, and the posterior distribution is Beta $(x+11, n-x+21)$. If the current experiment has 40 trials and 15 successes, the posterior distribution is Beta (26, 46) with mean 26/72 = .361, compared to a prior mean of .343. Figure 4.1 gives the posterior density of θ based on a histogram of 1000 θ values generated from the Beta (26,46) distribution. The author used Minitab to generate the θ values for the histogram.

Now, let us consider a random sample $x = (x_1, x_2, \quad, x_n)$ of size n from a normal $(\mu, 1/\tau)$ population, where $\tau = 1/\sigma^2$ is the inverse of the variance, and suppose the prior information is vague and the Jeffrey's prior $\xi(\mu, \tau) \propto 1/\tau$

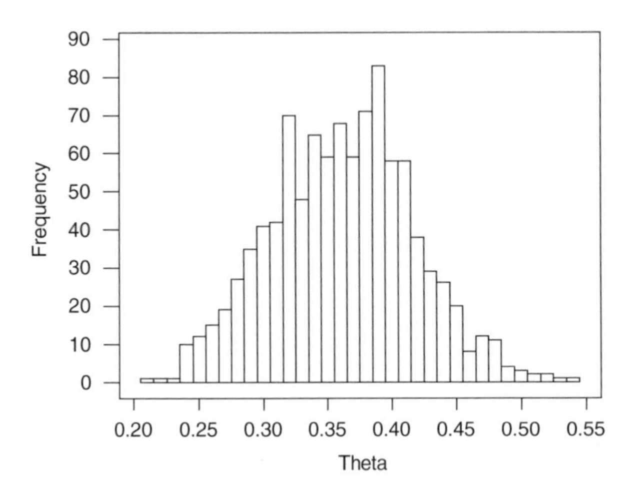

FIGURE 4.1
Posterior distribution of theta.

is appropriate, then the posterior density of the parameters is

$$\xi(\mu,\tau/x) \propto \tau^{n/2-1} \exp-(\tau/2)\left[n(\mu-\bar{x})^2 + \sum_{i=1}^{i=n}(x_i-\bar{x})^2 \right]. \tag{4.14}$$

Using the properties of the gamma density, τ is eliminated by integrating the joint density with respect to τ to give

$$\xi(\mu/x) = \{\Gamma(n/2)n^{1/2}/(n-1)^{1/2}$$

$$\times S\pi^{1/2}\Gamma((n-1)/2)\}/[1+n(\mu-\bar{x})^2/(n-1)S^2]^{(n-1+1)/2}, \tag{4.15}$$

which is recognized as a t distribution with $n - 1$ degrees of freedom, location $\bar{x}$ and precision n/S^2. Transforming to $(\mu-\bar{x})\sqrt{n}/S$, the resulting variable has a Student's t-distribution with $n - 1$ degrees of freedom. Note the mean of μ is the sample mean, while the variance is $[(n\text{-}1)/n(n\text{-}3)]S^2, n > 3$.

Eliminating μ from Equation (4.14) results in the marginal distribution of τ as

$$\xi(\tau/x) \propto \tau^{[(n-1)/2]-1} \exp-\tau(n-1)S^2/2 \text{ , } \tau > 0, \tag{4.16}$$

which is a gamma density with parameters $(n - 1)/2$ and $(n - 1)S^2/2$.

We return to the Carlin[21] example found in WinBUGS where the mortality of the treatment (beta blockers to prevent heart attack) and control groups is compared on the basis of a meta-analysis of 22 clinical trials.

TABLE 4.2

Posterior Distribution of Delta and Sigma

Parameter	Mean	Std. Dev.	Median	Lower	Upper
delta	–.2513	.061	–.2313.	–.3701	–.1265
sigma	.1143	.0672	.1020	.0265	.2731

The posterior analysis will be executed with the emphasis placed on the posterior distribution of delta, which measures the effect of the beta blocker treatment. If the effect is zero, beta blockers have no effect on mortality compared to the control groups. The program statements are given by Equation (4.12), and the analysis executed with 50,000 values generated from the posterior distributions of delta and sigma = 1/tau. The parameter d is the mean of the delta parameters, while sigma is the standard deviation, and both parameters are given noninformative prior distributions. The characteristics of the posterior distribution of delta and tau are given in Table 4.2.

The analysis also generates a graph of the posterior densities. See Figure 4.2 for the graph of the posterior distributions of d. Is there a treatment effect? The mass of the posterior distribution is to the left of zero where the lower $2\frac{1}{2}\%$ point is –.3701 and the upper –.1265, thus the posterior evidence suggests that delta is not zero on the logit scale and that beta blockers lower the mortality of a heart attack.

In Figure 4.3, one sees the posterior distribution of sigma is skewed to the right. This plot was done with the WinBUGS package. The actual execution of the simulation will be explained later in this chapter.

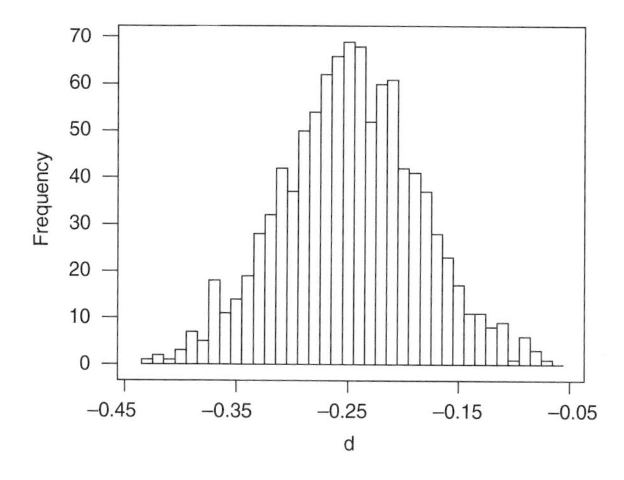

FIGURE 4.2
Posterior distribution of d.

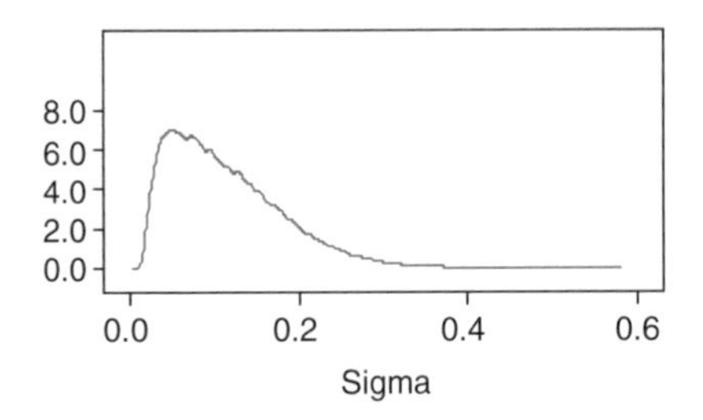

FIGURE 4.3
Posterior density of sigma.

4.5 Inference

4.5.1 Introduction

In a statistical context, "inference" usually means estimation of parameters, tests of hypotheses, and prediction of future observations. With the Bayesian approach, all inferences are based on the posterior distribution of the parameters, which in turn is based on the sample via the likelihood function and the prior distribution. We have seen the role of the prior and likelihood function in determining the posterior distribution, and presently we will focus on the determination of point and interval estimation of the model and, later, will concentrate on how the posterior distribution determines a test of hypothesis.

When a model has only one parameter, one would estimate that parameter by listing its characteristics, such as the posterior mean, media, and standard deviation, and plotting the posterior density. On the other hand, if there are several parameters, one would determine the marginal posterior distribution of the relevant parameters and, as above, calculate its characteristics (e.g., mean, median, mode, standard deviation, etc.) and plot the densities. Interval estimates of the parameters are also usually reported and are termed "credible" intervals.

4.5.2 Estimation

Suppose we want to estimate θ of the binomial example of the previous section, where the density is shown in Figure 4.1. The posterior distribution is Beta (21,46) with the following characteristics: mean = .361, median = .362, standard deviation = .055 lower $2\frac{1}{2}\%$ point = .254, and .473 = upper $2\frac{1}{2}\%$ point. The mean and median are the same as implied by the symmetry of the plot in Figure 4.1, while the lower and upper $2\frac{1}{2}\%$ points determine a 95% credible interval of (.254, .473) for θ.

Inferences for the normal (μ, τ) population are somewhat more demanding because both parameters are unknown. Assuming the vague prior density

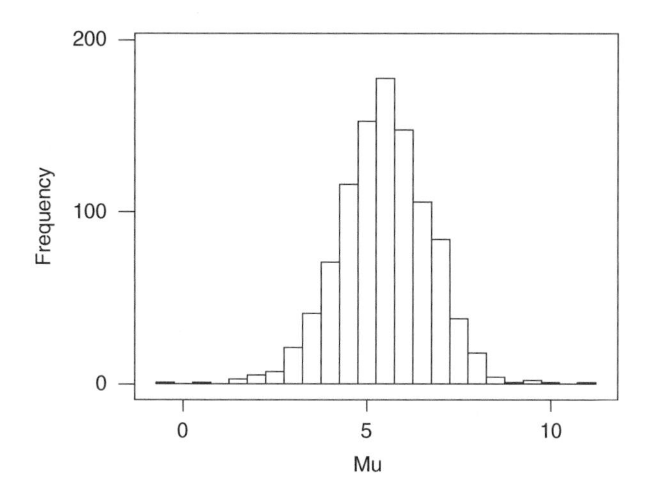

FIGURE 4.4
Posterior distribution of mu.

$\xi(\mu,\tau) \propto 1/\tau$, the marginal posterior distribution of the population mean μ is a t-distribution with $n - 1$ degrees of freedom, mean $\bar{x}$, and precision n/S^2 ($S^2$is the sample variance), thus the mean and the median are the same and provide a natural estimator of μ, and because of the symmetry of the t-density, a $(1 - \alpha)$ credible interval for μ is $\bar{x} \pm t_{\alpha/2,n-1} S/\sqrt{n}$ where $t_{\alpha/2,n-1}$ is the upper 100 $\alpha/2$% point of the t-distribution with $n - 1$ degrees of freedom. Suppose $n = 10$, $x = (1,2,3,4,5,6,7,8,9,10)$, $\bar{x} = 5.500$ and $S = 3.028$, then the histogram of 1000 values generated from the t (9, 5.5, 1.090) distribution is given in Figure 4.4. A 95% credible interval is $5.5 \pm .822\ (3.028)/3.162 = (4.713, 6.287)$. Using the same dataset, the following WinBUGS instructions below were used to analyze the problem.

```
model
{ for( i in 1:10) { x[i]~dnorm(mu,tau) }
mu~dnorm (0.0,.0001)
tau ~dgamma( .0001,.0001)                    (4.17)
sigma <- 1/tau }
list( x = c(1,2,3,4,5,6,7,8,9,10))
list( mu = 0, tau = 1)
```

Note that a somewhat different prior was employed here compared to previously, in that μ and τ are independent and assigned proper but noninformative distributions. The corresponding analysis is given in Table 4.3.

Upper and lower refer to the lower and upper $2\frac{1}{2}$% points of the posterior distribution. The plot of the posterior density of μ is the same as in Figure 4.4. The posterior density of sigma (Figure 4.5) shows the skewness to the right

TABLE 4.3

Posterior Distribution of μ and $\sigma = 1/\sqrt{\tau}$

Parameter	Mean	Std. Dev.	Median	Lower	Upper
mu	5.48	1.10	5.49	3.30	7.67
sigma	11.86	7.77	9.92	4.33	30.47

with a median of 9.92, a mean of 11.86 and a 95% credible interval of (4.33, 30.47).

The program generated 10,000 samples from the posterior distribution of μ using a Gibbs sampling algorithm, and one did not have to know the analytical form (e.g., a formula) for the posterior density.

4.5.3 Testing Hypotheses

4.5.3.1 Introduction

An important feature of inference is testing hypotheses. Often in accuracy studies, the scientific hypothesis of that study can be expressed in statistical terms and a formal test implemented. Suppose $\Omega = \Omega_0 \cup \Omega_1$ is a partition of the parameter space, then the null hypothesis is designated as H: $\theta \in \Omega_0$ and the alternative by A: $\theta \in \Omega_1$, and a test of H vs. A consists of rejecting H in favor of A if the observations $x = (x_1, x_2, \ldots, x_n)$ belong to a critical region C. In the usual approach, the critical region is based on the probabilities of type I errors, namely $Pr(C/\theta)$, where $\theta \in \Omega_0$, and of type II errors $1-Pr(C/\theta)$, where $\theta \in \Omega_1$. This approach to testing hypothesis was developed by Neyman and Pearson and can be found in many of the standard references, such as Lehmann.[22]

In the Bayesian approach, the decision to reject the null hypothesis is based on the probability of the alternative hypothesis

$$\varsigma_1 = Pr(\theta \in \Omega_1 / x), \tag{4.18}$$

and the probability of the null hypothesis

$$\varsigma_0 = Pr(\theta \in \Omega_0 / x).$$

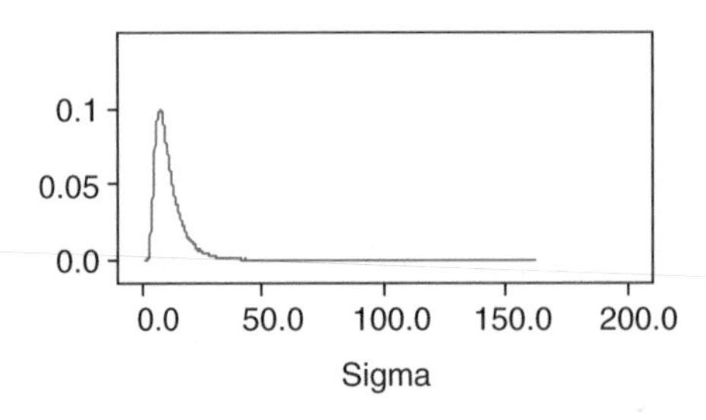

FIGURE 4.5
Density of sigma.

Thus, the larger the ς_1, the more the indication that H is false. If π_0 and π_1 denote the prior probabilities of the null and alternative hypotheses, respectively, the Bayes factor is defined as

$$B = (\varsigma_0 / \varsigma_1) / (\pi_0 / \pi_1), \tag{4.19}$$

where the numerator is the posterior odds of the null hypothesis relative to the alternative, and the denominator is the corresponding prior odds.

Suppose θ is scalar and that H: $\theta < \theta_0$ and A: $\theta > \theta_0$, where $\theta \in \Omega$, and Ω is a subset of the real numbers, then H and A are one-sided hypotheses. This situation can occur when there are so-called nuisance parameters in the model. For example, if θ is the mean of normal population, then the unknown standard deviation would be considered a nuisance parameter since the primary focus is on the mean.

On the other hand, suppose H: $\theta = \theta_0$ and A: $\theta \neq \theta_0$, then the alternative is two-sided, and the null is referred to as a sharp null hypothesis. Note, in this situation, θ can be multidimensional and nuisance parameters can be present. For a sharp null hypothesis, special attention to the prior must be given to the null hypothesis. Let π_0 denote the probability of the null hypothesis, let $\pi_1 = 1 - \pi_0$, and suppose $\pi_1 \xi_1(\theta)$ is the prior density of θ when $\theta \neq \theta_0$.

The marginal density of X is

$$f(x) = \pi_0 f(x / \theta_0) + \pi_1 f_1(x), \tag{4.20}$$

where

$$f_1(x) = \int_\Omega \xi_1(\theta) f(x / \theta) d\theta \ .$$

The posterior probabilities of the null and alternative hypotheses are

$$\varsigma_0 = [\pi_0 f(x / \theta_0)] / [\pi_0 f(x / \theta_0) + \pi_1 f_1(x)] \tag{4.21}$$

and $\varsigma_1 = 1 - \varsigma_0$, respectively.

4.5.3.2 Binomial Example of Testing

A binomial example is considered in the context of a Phase II clinical trial, where the null and alternative hypotheses are one-sided. Consider a random sample from a Bernoulli population with parameters n and θ, where n is the number of patients and θ is the probability of a response. Let X be the number of responses among n patients, and suppose the null hypothesis is H: $\theta \leq \theta_0$ vs. the alternative A: $\theta > \theta_0$. From previous related studies and the experience of the investigators, the prior information for θ is determined to be Beta (a,b), thus the posterior distribution of θ is Beta $(x + a, n - x + b)$, where x is the observed number of responses among n patients. The null hypothesis is rejected in favor of the alternative when

$$Pr[\theta > \theta_0 / \; x, n] > \gamma, \tag{4.22}$$

where γ is usually some "large" value as .90, .95, or .99. The above equation determines the critical region of the test, thus the power function is

$$g(\theta) = Pr_{X/\theta} \; \{Pr[\theta > \theta_0 / x, n] > \gamma\}, \tag{4.23}$$

where the outer probability is with respect to the conditional distribution of X given θ.

4.5.3.3 Comparing Two Binomial Populations

Comparing two binomial populations is a common problem in statistics and involves the null hypothesis H: $\theta_1 = \theta_2$ vs. the alternative A: $\theta_1 \neq \theta_2$, where θ_1 and θ_2 are parameters from two Bernoulli populations. The two Bernoulli parameters might be the sensitivities of two diagnostic modalities.

Assuming the prior probability of the null hypothesis is π and assigning independent uniform priors for the two Bernoulli parameters, it can be shown (see Equation 4.21) that the Bayesian test rejects H in favor of A if the posterior probability P of the alternative hypothesis satisfies

$$P > \gamma, \tag{4.24}$$

where

$$P = D_2 / D \tag{4.25}$$

and $D = D_1 + D_2$. It can be shown (see Equation 4.21) that

$$D_1 = \left\{ \pi \binom{n_1}{x_1} \binom{n_2}{x_2} \Gamma(x_1 + x_2 + 1) \Gamma(n_1 + n_2 - x_1 - x_2 + 1) \right\} \div \Gamma(n_1 + n_2 + 2) \tag{4.26}$$

where Γ is the gamma function.

Note that $D_2 = (1 - \pi)(n_1 + 1)^{-1} \, (n_2 + 1)^{-1}$, and π is the prior probability of the null hypothesis. X_1 and X_2 are the number of responses from the two binomial populations with parameters (θ_1, n_1) and (θ_2, n_2), respectively.

Note that the power function is given by

$$g(\theta_1, \theta_2) = Pr_{x_1, x_2 / \theta_1, \theta_2} \; [P > \gamma / \; x_1, x_2, n_1, n_2], \quad (\theta_1, \theta_2) \in (0,1) \times (0,1), \tag{4.27}$$

where P is given by Equation (4.25) and the outer probability is with respect to the conditional distribution of X_1 and X_2, given θ_1 and θ_2. This will be used for sample size calculations in the following section.

4.5.3.4 Sharp Null Hypothesis for the Normal Mean

Let $N(\theta, \tau^{-1})$ denote a normal population with mean θ and precision τ, where both are unknown and then suppose we want to test the null hypothesis $H: \theta = \theta_0$ vs. $A: \theta \neq \theta_0$, based on a random sample of size n with sample mean $\bar{x}$ and variance S^2. Assume the prior probability of the null hypothesis is α and a noninformative prior distribution

$$\xi(\theta, \tau) \propto 1/\tau$$

for θ and τ, then the Bayesian test is to reject the null in favor of the alternative if the posterior probability P of the alternative hypothesis satisfies

$$P > \gamma$$

where

$$P = D_2/D \tag{4.28}$$

and

$$D = D_1 + D_2.$$

It can be shown (see Equation 4.21) that

$$D_1 = \{\alpha\Gamma(n/2)2^{n/2}\}/\{(2\pi)^{n/2}\,[n(\theta_0 - \bar{x})^2 + (n-1)S^2]^{n/2}\}$$

and

$$D_2 = \{(1-\alpha)\Gamma((n-1)/2)\,2^{(n-1)/2}\}/\{(2\pi)^{(n-1)/2}[(n-1)S^2]^{(n-1)/2}\}$$

where α is the prior probability of the null hypothesis.

The above three examples involve standard one- and two-sample problems and will be applied in the context of diagnostic test accuracy and reader agreement studies and will be visited again when illustrating sample size estimation.

4.6 Sample Size

4.6.1 Introduction

When designing a study for diagnostic accuracy, one must take into consideration the reliability of the study. The more patients in the study, the more information is available for estimation and tests of hypotheses. The main focus will be in justifying the sample size to minimize the errors in testing hypotheses.

For example, suppose two imaging modalities (e.g., CT vs. MRI) for diagnosing lung cancer are to be compared on the basis of test accuracy (sensitivity, specificity, and the area under the ROC curve). How many patients are sufficient to reject the null hypothesis that the test accuracy is the same for both modalities in favor of the alternative that one has greater accuracy than the other? Such examples will be introduced in the next section using the one- and two-sample binomial studies of the previous section.

Suppose a Phase II clinical trial is to be designed where diagnostic imaging is monitoring the response of a solid tumor to therapy. In these cases, a sequential sampling plan, with stopping rules, is appropriate for testing the null hypothesis that the response rate is less than some predetermined value and below which the therapy would no longer be of interest. Bayesian sequential techniques that estimate the sample size and that determine stopping rules will be discussed in detail in Chapter 8.

4.6.2 A One-Sample Binomial for Response

The binomial example of Section 4.5.3.2 is revisited here where a clinical trial is considered with one-sided null and alternative hypotheses. Consider a random sample from a Bernoulli population with parameters n and θ, where n is the number of patients and θ is the probability of a response. Let X be the number of responses among n patients, and suppose the null hypotheses are H: $\theta \le \theta_0$ vs. the alternative A: $\theta > \theta_0$. From previous related studies and the experience of the investigators, the prior information for θ is determined to be Beta (a,b), thus the posterior distribution of θ is Beta $(x + a, n - x + b)$. The null hypothesis is rejected in favor of the alternative when

$$Pr[\theta > \theta_0/x, n] > \gamma$$

where γ is usually some "large" value as .90, .95, or .99. The above equation determines the critical region of the test, thus the power function of the test is

$$g(\theta) = Pr_{X/\theta}\{Pr[\theta > \theta_0/x, n] > \gamma\}$$

where the outer probability is with respect to the conditional distribution of X given θ.

The power (Equation 4.23) at a given value of θ is interpreted as a simulation as follows:

1. Select n and θ and set $I = 0$.
2. Generate $X \sim$ Binomial (θ, n).
3. Generate $\theta \sim$ Beta$(x + a, n - x + b)$.
4. If $Pr\,[\theta > \theta_0/x, n] > \gamma$, let the counter $I = I + 1$, otherwise let $I = I$. (4.29)

5. Repeat (1) – (4) M times, where M is "large."
6. Select another θ and repeat (2) – (5), then the power is estimated as I/M.

We consider a typical trial where the historical rate for response to therapy is .20, thus the trial is to be stopped if this rate exceeds the historical value. Response rates are carefully defined in the study protocol. The null and alternative hypotheses are given as

$$H: \theta \leq .20 \quad \text{and} \quad A: \theta > .20 \tag{4.30}$$

where θ is the response rate to therapy. The null hypothesis is rejected if the posterior probability of the alternative hypothesis is greater than the threshold value γ.

When a uniform prior is appropriate, the power curve for the following scenarios is computed (see Equation (4.23) and Equation (4.29)), with sample sizes $n = 125$, 205, and 500, threshold values $\gamma = .90, .95, .99$, $M = 1000$, and null value $\theta_0 = .20$. (See Table 4.4 below for the power of the test for various values of θ.)

Note that the power of the test at $\theta = .30$ and $\gamma = .95$ is .841, .958, and .999 for $N = 125$, 205, and 500, respectively.

The Bayesian test behaves in a reasonable way. For the conventional type I error of .05, a sample size of $N = 125$ would be sufficient to detect the difference .3 vs. .2 with a power of .841. On the other hand, in order to detect the alternative .4 with 125 patients, the power is essentially 1. To estimate the sample size for scenarios other than those given by the table, one must use the simulation (Equation (4.29)). When employing a conventional sample size program, such as PASS®, the power is .80 for detecting a response rate of .3, which is comparable to the .841 with the Bayesian simulation.

TABLE 4.4

Power Function for H vs. A, $N = 125,205,500$

	γ		
	.90	**.95**	**.99**
θ			
0	0,0,0	0,0,0	0,0,0
.1	0,0,0	0,0,0	0,0,0
.2	.107, .099, .08	.047, .051, .05	.013, .013, .008
.3	.897, .97,1	.841, .958, .999	.615, .82, .996
.4	1,1,1	1,1,1	.996,1,1
.5	1,1,1	1,1,1	1,1,1
.6	1,1,1	1,1,1	1,1,1
.7	1,1,1	1,1,1	1,1,1
.8	1,1,1	1,1,1	1,1,1
.9	1,1,1	1,1,1	1,1,1
1.0	1,1,1	1,1,1	1,1,1

4.6.3 One-Sample Binomial with Prior Information

Suppose we consider the same problem as above, but where prior information is available with 50 patients, 10 of who have responded to therapy. The null and alternative hypotheses are as above; however the null is rejected whenever

$$Pr[\theta > \phi/x, n] > \gamma \tag{4.31}$$

where θ is independent of $\phi \sim$ Beta (10,40). This can be considered as a two-sample problem where a future study is to be compared to a historical control. As above, using the simulation rules of Equation (4.29), the power function for the critical region (Equation (4.31)) is computed. (See Table 4.5 with the same sample sizes and threshold values as in Table 4.4.)

The power of the test is .758, .865, and .982 for $\theta = .4$, for $N = 125$, 205, and 500, respectively.

We see how important prior information is for testing hypotheses. If the hypothesis is rejected with the critical region

$$Pr[\theta > .2/x, n] > \gamma, \tag{4.32}$$

the power (see Table 4.4) will be larger than the corresponding power (see Table 4.5) determined by the critical region (Equation (4.31)) because of the additional variability introduced by the historical information contained in ϕ. Thus, larger sample sizes are required with the approach (Equation (4.31)) to achieve the same power as with the test given by Equation (4.32). On the other hand, if the prior information is incorporated directly into the likelihood function, the power function is higher for all values of θ, because of the increased sample size. Of course, if this is done, one is ignoring the prior variability of the historical control.

TABLE 4.5

Power for One-Sample Binomial with Prior Information

	γ		
θ	**.90**	**.95**	**.99**
0	0,0,0	0,0,0	0,0,0
.1	0,0,0	0,0,0	0,0,0
.2	.016, .001, .000	.002, .000, .000	.000, .000, .000
.3	.629, .712, .850	.362, .374, .437	.004, .026, .011
.4	.996, .999,1	.973, .998,1	*.758, .865, .982
.5	1,1,1	1,1,1	.999,1,1
.6	1,1,1	1,1,1	1,1,1
.7	1,1,1	1,1,1	1,1,1
.8	1,1,1	1,1,1	1,1,1
.9	1,1,1	1,1,1	1,1,1
1.0	1,1,1	1,1,1	1,1,1

TABLE 4.6

Power for Two-Sample Binomial

	θ_2									
	.1	.2	.3	.4	.5	.6	.7	.8	.9	1
θ_1										
.1	.004	.032	.135	.360	.621	.842	.958	.992	1	1
.2	.031	.011	.028	.106	.281	.536	.744	.913	.997	1
.3	.171	.028	.006	.029	.107	.252	.487	.767	.961	1
.4	.368	.098	.025	.013	.028	.075	.244	.542	.847	.999
.5	.619	.289	.100	.022	.007	.017	.108	.291	.640	.981
.6	.827	.527	.237	.086	.035	.005	.027	.116	.357	.882
.7	.950	.775	.464	.254	.113	.037	.013	.049	.171	.587
.8	.996	.928	.768	.491	.316	.132	.028	.010	.040	.205
.9	1	.996	.946	.840	.647	.359	.156	.037	.006	.014
1	1	1	1	1	.984	.873	.567	.200	.017	.000

4.6.4 Comparing Two Binomial Populations

The case of two binomial populations was introduced in Section 4.5.3.3 where Equation (4.27) determines the power function for testing H: $\theta_1 = \theta_2$ vs. the alternative A: $\theta_1 \neq \theta_2$. The power function of the test at (θ_1, θ_2) is

$$g(\theta_1,\theta_2) = Pr_{x_1,x_2/\theta_1,\theta_2}\,[P > \gamma / x_1, x_2, n_1, n_2], \quad (\theta_1,\theta_2) \in (0,1) \times (0,1).$$

Suppose $n_1 = 20 = n_2$ are the sample sizes of the two groups and the prior probability of the null hypotheses is .5. The power at each point (θ_1, θ_2) is calculated via simulation, similar to that given by Equation (4.12) with $\gamma = .90$. The values are given in Table 4.6.

When the power is calculated with PASS for the two-sample, two-tailed binomial test with alpha = .013, sample sizes $n_1 = 20 = n_2$, and $(\theta_1, \theta_2) = (.3, .9)$, the power is .922, which is less than the power of the Bayesian test. Adjustments in γ of the Bayesian test would give a power equal to that of the conventional test. For the θ_1 and θ_2 values considered, the maximum type I error for the Bayesian test is approximately .013.

4.7 Computing

4.7.1 Introduction

This section introduces the computing algorithms and software that will be used for the Bayesian analysis of problems in diagnostic accuracy. In the previous sections, direct methods of computing the characteristics of the posterior distribution were demonstrated with some standard one-sample and two-sample problems. An example of this is the posterior analysis of a

TABLE 4.7

Distribution of Patients for Test Accuracy

	Disease Status		
New Test	$D = 0$	$D = 1$	Row Total
X = 0	n_{00}	n_{01}	$n_{0.}$
X = 1	n_{10}	n_{11}	$n_{1.}$
Column Total	$n_{.0}$	$n_{.1}$	

binomial population (Equation (4.13)), where the posterior distribution of θ was Beta and samples were generated from its posterior distribution by a random number generator in Minitab.

Also, MCMC techniques for sampling from the posterior distribution were illustrated by comparing the mortality of beta blockers for prevention of heart attacks with the control group. The WinBUGS statements are listed in Equation (4.12), and the analysis consisted of plotting the posterior density of the parameter that measures the effect of treatment on mortality.

4.7.2 Direct Methods of Computation

To illustrate the direct method for the Bayesian analysis of a problem, the accuracy of a binary test is considered. How well does the test differentiate between diseased and nondiseased patients? Consider Table 4.7 that classifies patients by disease status negative or positive, ($D = 0$ or $D = 1$), and the results of a new diagnostic test as negative or positive ($X = 0$ or $X = 1$). (See Jarvik[23] for additional details on binary tests for accuracy of diagnostic procedures.)

Suppose the patients are classified by disease status and by the outcome of a new diagnostic test, with the results given by Table 4.8, and let the corresponding joint probabilities of disease and test results be given as in the table.

The probability that a nondiseased patient will have a negative test (a true negative (TN)) is $P(X = 0, D = 0) = \theta_{00}$; the probability that a patient will have a positive test results is $P(X = 1) = \theta_{1.}$; and the probability of a true positive (TP) is $P(X = 1, D = 1) = \theta_{11}$, etc.

If the patients are selected at random from the population, the disease incidence is $P(D = 1) = \theta_{.1}$. In order to perform a Bayesian determination of test accuracy, a prior probability density must be assigned to the parameters,

TABLE 4.8

Joint Probabilities of Disease Status and Test Results

	Disease Status		
New Test	$D = 0$	$D = 1$	Row Total
X = 0	θ_{00}(TN)	θ_{01}(FN)	$\theta_{0.}$
X = 1	θ_{10} (FP)	θ_{11}(TP)	$\theta_{1.}$
Column Total	$\theta_{.0}$	$\theta_{.1}$	

TABLE 4.9

Results of Diagnostic Test

	Disease Status		
New Test	$D = 0$	$D = 1$	**Row Total**
$X = 0$	90	10	100
$X = 1$	10	90	100
Column Total	100	100	200

which when combined with the likelihood function

$$L(\theta/n) \propto \theta_{00}^{n_{00}}\theta_{01}^{n_{01}}\theta_{10}^{n_{10}}\theta_{11}^{n_{11}}$$

via the Bayes theorem, yields the posterior density. The parameter $\theta = (\theta_{00}, \theta_{01}, \theta_{10}, \theta_{11})$ is the vector of unknown parameters, and the likelihood function is based on the joint multinomial distribution of $n = (n_{00}, n_{01}, n_{10}, n_{11})$ of the number of patients in each category, given θ. If a uniform prior density is appropriate, the joint density of the parameters is

$$\xi(\theta / n) = \{\Gamma(n_{00} + n_{01} + n_{10} + n_{11}) / \Gamma(n_{00})\Gamma(n_{01})\Gamma(n_{10})\Gamma(n_{11})\}\theta_{00}^{n_{00}}\theta_{01}^{n_{01}}\theta_{10}^{n_{10}}\theta_{11}^{n_{11}}, \quad (4.33)$$

where $0 \le \theta_{ij} \le 1$ and $\Sigma_{i=0}^{i=1}\Sigma_{j=0}^{j=1}\theta_{ij} = 1$. Therefore $\theta \sim \text{Dir}\,(n_{00} + 1, n_{01} + 1, n_{10} + 1, n_{11} + 1)$, a Dirichlet distribution, and all inferences will be based on it.

Suppose the results of the diagnostic test are given by Table 4.9.

How is test accuracy estimated? For example, what is the estimated sensitivity

$$P(X = 1/D = 1) = \theta_{11} / (\theta_{01} + \theta_{11})\ ? \quad (4.34)$$

Minitab is used to directly sample from the posterior distribution of the four parameters of the Dirichlet as follows:

1. Generate 1000 values from the joint distribution of $(\theta_{00}, \theta_{01}, \theta_{10}, \theta_{11})$. This will produce four columns of Dirichlet values in the worksheet. For the fifth column, calculate the sensitivity $\theta_{11} / (\theta_{01} + \theta_{11})$.
2. Calculate the descriptive statistics (mean, median, standard deviation) for the 1000 sensitivity values of the fifth column.
3. Estimate the lower and upper $2\frac{1}{2}$ percentiles from the sorted 1000 sensitivity values.
4. Plot the histogram of the sensitivity values.

In a similar way, the positive predictive value

$$P(D = 1/X = 1) = \theta_{11} / (\theta_{10} + \theta_{11}) \quad (4.35)$$

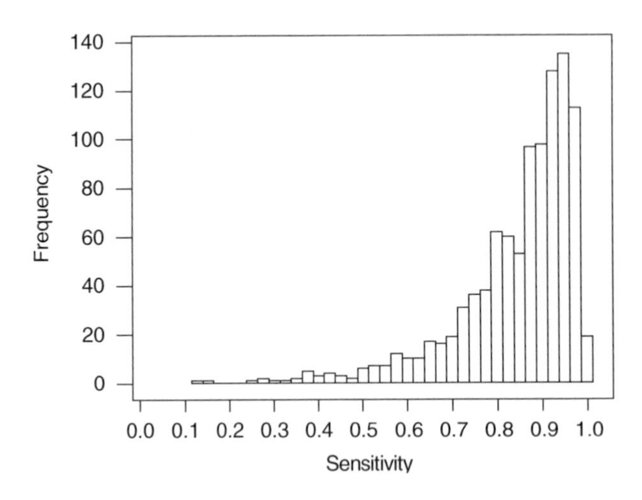

FIGURE 4.6
Histogram of the sensitivity.

is estimated with a posterior mean = .489, median = .886, sd = .136, and 95% credible interval (.477, .989), and as with the sensitivity, has a posterior distribution, which is skewed to the left. The histogram of 1000 values generated from the marginal posterior distribution of the sensitivity shows the skewness (Figure 4.6). Other measures of accuracy include the specificity $\theta_{00} / (\theta_{00} + \theta_{10})$, and the negative predictive value

$$P(D=0/X=0) = \theta_{00} / (\theta_{00} + \theta_{01}).$$

Direct sampling will be used frequently for the more elementary problems in diagnostic accuracy and Minitab® can be downloaded at *www.minitab.com* The WinBUGS program below will execute the same analysis as Minitab.

```
model;
{
  g00 ~dgamma(a00,b00);
  g01 ~dgamma(a01,b01);
  g10 ~dgamma(a10,b10);
  g11 ~dgamma(a11,b11);
  h<- g00+g01+g10+g11;

  theta00<-g00/h
  theta01<-g01/h
  theta10<-g10/h
  theta11<-g11/h
```

```
# the theta are those in Table 4.8
sen<-theta11/(theta01+theta11)
# sen is the sensitivity
ppv<- theta11/(theta10+theta11)
# ppv is the positive predictive value
}
list( a00 =91, b00 = 2, a01 = 11, b01 = 2, a10 =11,
b10 = 2, a11 = 91, b11 = 2)
list( g00 = 2, g01=2,g10=2,g11=2)
```

The program uses the same approach as Minitab to calculate the sensitivity and specificity, namely DeGroot[24], p. 63, prob. 5. The notation used mimics that of Table 4.8 and Equation (4.34) and Equation (4.35). More details on executing this program are described in the following sections.

4.7.3 Gibbs Sampling

4.7.3.1 Introduction

The direct sampling approach described above will be used frequently; however it has some limitations. For example, when considering a hierarchical model with many levels of parameters, it is more appropriate to use an MCMC technique in order to sample from the many posterior distributions. Gibbs sampling can be thought of as a practical way to implement the fact that the joint distribution of two random variables is determined by the two conditional distributions.

The two variable cases are considered first by starting with a pair (θ_1,θ_2) of random variables. The Gibbs sampler generates a random sample from the joint distribution of θ_1 and θ_2 by sampling from the conditional distributions of θ_1, given θ_2, and from θ_2, given θ_1. The Gibbs sequence of size k

$$\theta_2^0,\theta_1^0;\theta_2^1,\theta_1^1;\theta_2^2,\theta_1^2;\ldots;\theta_2^k,\theta_1^k \tag{4.36}$$

is generated by first choosing the initial values θ_2^0,θ_1^0, while the remaining are obtained iteratively by alternating values from the two conditional distributions. Under quite general conditions, for large enough k, the final two values θ_2^k,θ_1^k are samples from their respective marginal distributions. To generate a random sample of size n from the joint posterior distribution, generate the above Gibbs sequence n times. Having generated values from the marginal distributions with large k and n, the sample mean and variance will converge to the corresponding mean and variance of the posterior distribution of (θ_1,θ_2).

Gibbs sampling is an example of an MCMC because the generated samples are drawn from the limiting distribution of a 2×2 Markov chain. (See Casella and George[25] for proof that the generated values are indeed values from the appropriate marginal distributions.) Of course, Gibbs sequences can be generated from the joint distribution of three, four, and more random variables.

The Gibbs sampling scheme is illustrated with three random variables for the common normal mean problem.

4.7.3.2 Common Mean of Normal Populations

Gregurich and Broemeling[26] describe the various steps in Gibbs sampling to determine the posterior distribution of the parameters in independent normal populations with a common mean.

In situations where the integration of the joint density is extremely difficult, an algorithm known as the Gibbs sampler has proven to be a good alternative. The Gibbs sampler generates a sample from the joint density by sampling instead from the conditional densities, which are often known. According to Casella and George, by generating a large enough sample, characteristics of the marginal density and even the density itself can be obtained. Since the conditional posterior distributions are easily obtained, the Gibbs sampling method will be used.

The Gibbs sampling approach can be best explained by illustrating the procedure using two normal populations with a common mean θ. Thus, let $y_{ij}, j=1,2,\ldots,n_i$ be a random sample of size n_i from a normal population for $i=1,2$.

The likelihood function for $\theta, \tau_1, and\ \tau_2$ is

$$L(\theta,\tau_1,\tau_2/data) \propto \tau_1^{\frac{n_1}{2}} \exp-\frac{\tau_1}{2}\left[(n_1-1)s_1^2+n_1(\theta-\bar{y}_1)^2\right] * \tau_2^{\frac{n_2}{2}} \exp$$

$$-\frac{\tau_2}{2}\left[(n_2-1)s_2^2+n_2(\theta-\bar{y}_2)^2\right]$$

where

$$\theta \in \Re, \quad \tau_1>0, \tau_2>0\ , \quad s_1^2=\sum_{j=1}^{n_1}(y_{1j}-\bar{y}_1)^2/(n_1-1)$$

and

$$s_2^2=\sum_{j=1}^{n_2}(y_{2j}-\bar{y}_2)^2/(n_2-1).$$

The prior distribution for the parameters $\theta, \tau_1, and\ \tau_2$ is assumed to be a vague prior defined as

$$g(\theta,\tau_1,\tau_2) \propto \frac{1}{\tau_1}\frac{1}{\tau_2}, \quad \tau_i>0.$$

Then, combining the above gives the posterior density of the parameters as

$$p(\theta,\tau_1,\tau_2\,/\,data) \propto \prod_{i=1}^{2} \tau_i^{\frac{n_i-1}{2}}\, exp - \frac{\tau_i}{2}\left[(n_i-1)s_i^2 + n_i(\theta-\bar{y}_i)^2\right].$$

Therefore, the conditional posterior distribution of τ_1 and τ_2, given θ, is

$$\tau_i/\theta \sim \text{Gamma}\left[\frac{n_i}{2}, \frac{(n_i-1)s_i^2 + n_i(\theta-\bar{y}_i)^2}{2}\right], \tag{4.37}$$

for i = 1, 2 and τ_1/θ and τ_2/θ are independent.

The conditional posterior distribution of θ given τ_1 and τ_2 is normal. It can be shown that

$$\theta/\tau_1,\tau_2 \sim N\left[\frac{n_1\tau_1\bar{y}_1 + n_2\tau_2\bar{y}_2}{n_1\tau_1 + n_2\tau_2}, (n_1\tau_1 + n_2\tau_2)^{-1}\right]. \tag{4.38}$$

Given the starting values $\tau_1^{(0)}, \tau_2^{(0)}, and\ \theta^{(0)}$ where

$$\tau_1^{(0)} = 1/s_1^2,$$

$$\tau_2^{(0)} = 1/s_2^2,$$

and

$$\theta^{(0)} = \frac{n_1\bar{y}_1 + n_2\bar{y}_2}{n_1 + n_2},$$

draw $\theta^{(1)}$ from the normal conditional distribution of θ, given $\tau_1 = \tau_1^{(0)}$ $and\ \tau_2 = \tau_2^{(0)}$. Then draw $\tau_1^{(1)}$ from the conditional gamma distribution, given $\theta = \theta^{(1)}$. And, lastly, draw $\tau_2^{(1)}$ from the conditional gamma distribution of τ_2, given $\theta = \theta^{(1)}$. Then generate

$$\theta^{(2)} \sim \theta/\tau_1 = \tau_1^{(1)}, \tau_2 = \tau_2^{(1)}$$

$$\tau_1^{(2)} \sim \tau_1/\theta = \theta^{(2)}$$

$$\tau_2^{(2)} \sim \tau_2/\theta = \theta^{(2)}.$$

Continue this process until there are t-iterations $(\theta^{(t)}, \tau_1^{(t)}, \tau_2^{(t)})$. For large t, $\theta^{(t)}$ would be one sample from the marginal distribution of θ, $\tau_1^{(t)}$ from the marginal distribution of τ_1, and $\tau_2^{(t)}$ from the marginal distribution of τ_2.

Independently repeating the above Gibbs process m times produces m 3-tuple parameter values $(\theta_j^{(t)}, \tau_{1j}^{(t)}, \tau_{2j}^{(t)}), j = 1,2,\ldots,m$, which represents a random sample of size m from the joint posterior distribution of (θ, τ_1, τ_2). The statistical inferences are drawn from the m sample values generated by the Gibbs sampler.

The statistical inferences can be drawn from the m sample values generated by the Gibbs sampler. The Gibbs sampler will produce four columns of samples (Table 4.10). Each row is a sample drawn from the posterior distribution of (θ, τ_1, τ_2). The first column is the sequence of the sample m, the second column is a random sample of size m from the poly-t-distribution of θ, and the third and fourth columns are also random samples of size m, but from the marginal posterior distributions of τ_1 *and* τ_2, respectively.

To obtain the characteristics of the marginal posterior distribution of a parameter, such as the mean and variance, it should be noted that the Gibbs sampler generates a sample of values of a marginal distribution from the conditional distributions without the actual marginal distribution. By simulating a large enough sample, the characteristics of the marginal can be calculated. If m is "large," the sample mean of the column of θs is

$$E(\theta/data) = \sum_{j=1}^{m} \theta_j^t / m = \bar{\theta}$$

thus, the mean of the posterior distribution of θ. The sample variance

$$(m-1)^{-1} \sum_{j=1}^{m} \left[\theta_j^t - \bar{\theta}\right]^2$$

is the variance of the posterior distribution of θ.

Additional characteristics, such as the median, mode, and the 95% credible region of the posterior distribution of the parameter θ, can be calculated from the samples generated by the Gibbs technique. Hypothesis testing can also be performed. Similar characteristics of the parameters τ_1 and τ_2 can be calculated from the samples resulting from the Gibbs method.

TABLE 4.10

Random Samples from Posterior Distribution

#	θ	τ_1	τ_2
1	θ_1^t	τ_{11}^t	τ_{21}^t
2	θ_2^t	τ_{21}^t	τ_{22}^t
…	…	…	…
m	θ_m^t	τ_{1m}^t	τ_{2m}^t

TABLE 4.11

Results from Gibbs Sampling

m	Mean	Standard Error Mean	95% Credible Interval
250	108.42	.07	106.03, 110.65
500	108.31	.04	106.35, 110.21
750	108.31	.03	106.64, 110.15
1500	108.36	.02	106.51, 110.26

The example is from Box and Tiao[12], p. 481. It is referred to as "the weighted mean problem." It has two sets of normally distributed independent samples with a common mean and different variances. Samples from the posterior distributions were generated from Gibbs sequences using the statistical software Minitab. The final value of each sequence was used to approximate the marginal posterior distribution of the parameters θ, τ_1 and τ_2. All Gibbs sequences were generated holding the value of t equal to 50. Each example has the results of the parameters using four different Gibbs sampler sizes where the sample size m is equal to 250, 500, 750, and 1500.

The "weighted mean problem" has two sets of normally distributed independent observations with a common mean, but different variances. The estimated values of θ determined by the Gibbs sampling method are shown in Table 4.11. The mean value of the posterior distribution of θ generated from the 250 Gibbs sequences is 108.42, with 0.07 the standard error of the mean. The mean value of θ generated from 500 and 750 Gibbs sequences have the same value of 108.31, and the standard errors of the mean equal 0.04 and 0.03, respectively. The mean value of θ generated from 1500 Gibbs sequences is 108.36 and a standard error of the mean of 0.02. Box and Tiao determined the posterior distribution of θ using an approximation approach. They estimated the value of θ to be 108.43. This is close to the value generated using the Gibbs sampler method. The exact posterior distribution of θ is the poly-t distribution. The effect of m appears to be minimal indicating that 500 to 750 iterations of the Gibbs sequence are sufficient.

4.7.3.3 MCMC Sampling with WinBUGS

The real power of MCMC techniques is when the posterior analysis is based on a hierarchical model that has several levels of parameters. The Carlin[21] example is revisited and is described in the help section of volume I of version 1.4 of the users manual, and the advantages of MCMC techniques are shown. The example was provided to illustrate a Bayesian posterior analysis in Section 4.3, and the program statements and worksheet are given below:

```
model
{
for( i in 1 : Num ) {
rc[i] ~ dbin(pc[i], nc[i])
rt[i] ~ dbin(pt[i], nt[i])
logit(pc[i]) <- m[i]
logit(pt[i]) <- m[i] + d[i]                              (4.12)
m[i] ~ dnorm(0.0,1.0E-5)
d[i] ~ dnorm(delta, tau)
}
delta ~ dnorm(0.0,1.0E-6)
tau ~ dgamma(0.001,0.001)

Data

list(rt = c(3, 7, 5, 102, 28, 4, 98, 60, 25, 138, 64,
45, 9, 57, 25, 33, 28, 8, 6, 32, 27, 22 ),
nt = c(38, 114, 69, 1533, 355, 59, 945, 632, 278,1916,
873, 263, 291, 858, 154, 207, 251, 151, 174, 209, 391,
680),
rc = c(3, 14, 11, 127, 27, 6, 152, 48, 37, 188, 52, 47,
16, 45, 31, 38, 12, 6, 3, 40, 43, 39),
nc = c(39, 116, 93, 1520, 365, 52, 939, 471, 282, 1921,
583, 266, 293, 883, 147, 213, 122, 154, 134, 218, 364,
674),
Num = 22)

Inits

list(delta = 0, d.new = 0, tau=1, m = c(0, 0, 0, 0, 0,
0, 0, 0, 0, 0, 0, 0, 0, 0, 0, 0, 0, 0, 0, 0, 0, 0),
d = c(0, 0, 0, 0, 0, 0, 0, 0, 0, 0, 0, 0, 0, 0, 0, 0,
0, 0, 0, 0, 0, 0))
```

TABLE 4.12

Gibbs Sampling with WinBUGS

Parameter	Mean	sd	MC Error	2.5%	Median	97.5%
delta	–.2489	.06282	.02297	–.3734	–.248	–.1239
tau	254	424.9	20.98	13.12	94.59	1511

This is a meta analysis that combines the information from 22 clinical trials that compare the mortality of the treatment group with a corresponding control group. The above statements are interpreted as follows.

Table 4.1 indicates that there are 38 patients in the treatment group of the first trial with 3 deaths compared to 3 deaths among 39 patients in the control group.

The worksheet above shows how the dataset is represented under the label "Data" with four columns: (1) the rt column listing the number of deaths in the 22 trials of the treatment group, (2) the nt column is the number of patients in the 22 trials of the treatment group, (3) the rc column is the number of deaths in the 22 control group trials, and (4) the nc the number of patients in the 22 control group trials. The Num = 22 is the number of clinical trials in the meta analysis.

The MCMC technique is iterative and initial values are required to begin the generation of the sequences. The initial values appear under the label "Inits," thus delta = 0, tau = 1 are the initial values of the delta and tau parameters, respectively, while 22 initial values (i.e., zeroes) are required for the m_i and d_i. The program is executed as follows:

1. Using the specification tool of the model menu: Click on the model menu and select the specification tool. Click on the word model at the beginning of the program statements, then click on check model box of the specification tool and the response should be "model is syntactically correct." Then click on the list statement in the worksheet, which appears to the right of the Data label, then click load data on the specification tool. Click on compile box of the specification tool and the response should be "model compiled." Lastly, click on Inits box of the specification tool and click on the word list, which appears to the right of the label Inits of the worksheet, and the response will be "model initialized."
2. To execute the program, bring down the model menu again and click on the updates icon. For the updates box, put the number of samples to be generated, say 10,000, and put, say, 100 for the length of the sequence in the refresh box.
3. Bring down the inference menu, and click on sample monitors tool. This will specify what parameters are to estimated. In the node box, type delta and click on set, then type tau in the node box and click on set, then type * in the node box. You are now ready to generate 10,000 samples from the marginal posterior distributions of delta and tau.
4. Return to the updates tool and click on the updates box. This executes the program.
5. In the samples monitor tool, click on stats, and the descriptive statistics (mean, sd, mc error, 2½%, median, 97.5%) from the posterior distribution are displayed. The outcomes are given above under the Results section of the worksheet.

For an experienced user of the software, the above actions will be familiar and easy to do; however, for the novice, it will appear somewhat confusing. The software requires some experience and the beginner can download WinBUGS at www.mrc-bsu.cam.ac.uk/bugs. The download will have a users manual and a very useful help menu, where many examples are provided that will be of invaluable assistance to the new user. Another good reference for using this software is Appendix B of Woodworth.[27]

4.8 Exercises

4.1. For the Beta density with parameters α and β, show that the mean is $[\alpha/(\alpha+\beta)]$ and the variance is $[\alpha\beta/(\alpha+\beta)^2(\alpha+\beta+1)]$.

4.2. From Equation (4.11), show the following: If the normal distribution is parameterized with μ and the precision $\tau = 1/\sigma^2$, the conjugate distribution is as follows: (1) the conditional distribution of μ, given τ, is normal with mean $\bar{x}$ and precision mτ, and (2) the marginal distribution of τ is gamma with parameters $(m-1)/2$ and $\Sigma_{i=1}^{i=m}(x_i-\bar{x})^2/2 = (m-1)S^2/2$, where S^2 is the sample variance.

4.3. Verify Table 4.2.

4.4. Verify the following statement : To generate values from the $t(n-1, \bar{x}, n/S^2)$ distribution, generate values from Student's *t*-distribution with $n-1$ degrees of freedom and multiply each by $\sqrt{n}/S$ and then add $\bar{x}$.

4.5: Verify Table 4.3.

4.6. Derive Equation (4.20) and Equation (4.21).

4.7. Verify Equation (4.23).

4.8. Describe the simulation used to compute the power (Equation (4.27)) for Table 4.4.

4.9. Verify that the descriptive statistics for the posterior distribution of the sensitivity are: posterior mean = .84, median = .89, sd = .133, lower $2\frac{1}{2}$% = .461, and upper $2\frac{1}{2}$% = .9842. The histogram of the sensitivity values is shown in Figure 4.6 and reflects the left skewness, which is shown by the median of .89, compared to a mean of .84. The maximum likelihood estimate is .90, with a standard deviation of .03. (See Equation (4.34) and Table 4.9.)

4.10. Verify Equation (4.37) and Equation (4.38).

4.12. Refer to Equation (4.38) and derive the marginal density of θ (the common mean of two normal populations).

4.13. Write a WinBUGS program and compute the posterior distribution of the common mean appearing in Table 4.11. Compare the results with those given by Minitab in Table 4.11.

4.14. See the results section of the WinBUGS program (Equation (4.12)). Verify the results of the posterior analysis of delta and tau using the statements in the program and the description for executing the program.

References

1. Bayes, T., An essay towards solving a problem in the doctrine of chances, *Philo. Trans. Roy. Soc. London*, 53, 370, 1764.
2. Laplace, P.S., *Memorie sur la probabilite de causes per les evenemens, Memories de l'Academie royale des sciences presentes par divers savans*, 1774, 621.
3. Laplace, P.S., *Memorie des les probabilities, Memories de l'Academie des sciences de Paris*, 1778, 227.
4. Stigler, M., The history of statistics. *The Measurement of Uncertainty before 1900*, The Belknap Press of Harvard University Press, Cambridge, MA, 1986.
5. Hald, A.A., *A History of Mathematical Statistics from 1750-1930*, Wiley Interscience, 1990, London.
6. Hald, A.A., *History of Mathematical Statistics before 1750*, Wiley Interscience, 1998, London.
7. Lhoste, E., *Le calcul des probabilites appliqué a l'artillerie, lois de probabilite a prior, Revu d'artillirie*, Mai, 405, 1923.
8. Jeffreys, H., *An Introduction to Probability*, Clarendon Press, 1939, Oxford, U.K.
9. Savage, L.J, *The Foundation of Statistics*, John Wiley & Sons, 1954, New York.
10. Lindley, D.V., *Introduction to Probability and Statistics from a Bayesian Viewpoint*, Vol. I and II, Cambridge University Press, 1965, Cambridge, U.K.
11. Broemeling, L.D and Broemeling, A.L., Studies in the history of probability and statistics XLVIII: the Bayesian contributions of Ernest Lhoste, *Biometrika*, 90(3),728, 2003.
12. Box, G.E.P. and Tiao, G.C., *Bayesian Inference in Statistical Analysis*, Addison Wesley, 1973, Reading, MA.
13. Zellner, A., *An Introduction to Bayesian Inference in Econometrics*, John Wiley & Sons, 1971, New York.
14. Broemeling, L.D., *The Bayesian Analysis of Linear Models*, Marcel Dekker, 1985, New York.
15. Leonard, T. and Hsu, J.S.J., Bayesian Methods. *An Analysis for Statisticians and Interdisciplinary Researchers*, Cambridge University Press, 1999, Cambridge, U.K.
16. Gelman, A., Carlin, J.B., Stern, H.S., and Rubin, D.B., *Bayesian Data Analysis*, Chapman & Hall/CRC, 1997, Boca Raton, FL.
17. Congdon, P., *Bayesian Statistical Modeling*, John Wiley & Sons, 2001, London.
18. Congdon, P., *Applied Bayesian Modeling*, John Wiley & Sons, 2003, New York.
19. Congdon, P., *Bayesian Models for Categorical Data*, John Wiley & Sons, 2005, New York.
20. Carlin, B.P. and Louis, T.A., *Bayes and Empirical Bayes for Data Analysis*, Chapman & Hall, 1996, New York.
21. Carlin, B.P., Taken from the Help Section of Vol. I of WinBUGS version 1.4, January 2003, Blocker: Random affects meta analysis of clinical trials.
22. Lehmann, E.L., *Testing Statistical Hypotheses*, John Wiley & Sons, 1959, New York.

23. Jarvik, G.J. Fundamentals of clinical research for radiologists. The research framework, *Am. J. Roentgenol.*, 176, 873, 2001.
24. DeGroot, M.H., *Optimal Statistical Decisions*, McGraw-Hill, 1970, New York.
25. Casella, G. and George, E.I., Explaining the Gibbs sampler, *Am. Stat.*, 46, 167, 1992.
26. Gregurich, M.A., and Broemeling, L.D., A Bayesian analysis for estimating the common mean of independent normal populations using the Gibbs sampler, *Commun. Stat. Theor. Meth.*, 26 (1), 25, 1997.
27. Woodworth, G.G., *Biostatistics, a Bayesian Introduction*, Wiley Interscience, 2005, Hoboken, NJ.

Chapter 5

Bayesian Methods for Diagnostic Accuracy

5.1 Introduction

This chapter describes the methodology for making inferences with respect to the basic measures of test accuracy and will begin with a section on the design of such studies. The elements of good design will be explained in the context of a protocol submission of a trial to assess the accuracy of a diagnostic test in a clinical situation. The submission procedure at the MD Anderson Cancer Center (MDACC) is very formal and all submissions are required to contain evidence of a well-designed experiment. The first step in protocol submission is the review by the Department of Biostatistics and Applied Mathematics.

After describing the components of designing a diagnostic study, this chapter introduces Bayesian methods for the analysis of diagnostic test accuracy, including the estimation of sensitivity, specificity, positive and negative predictive values, positive and negative diagnostic likelihood ratios, and receiving operating characteristic (ROC) curves. A Bayesian analysis determines the posterior distribution of the relevant parameter and its characteristics, such as the posterior mean, median, standard deviation, credible intervals, and associated plots of the density.

The analysis of test accuracy data is introduced first with binary and ordinal diagnostic test data, and then the Bayesian analysis is repeated with quantitative scores. Various imaging modalities are compared in a Bayesian framework by testing hypotheses, such as that one modality has greater accuracy (e.g., sensitivity or ROC area) than another, or that two modalities have equivalent accuracy.

This is followed by more specialized topics including localization and detection of disease by diagnostic tests where the image is partitioned into regions of interest (ROI). This is interesting statistically because of the correlation between regions of the same image are correlated. The analysis of correlated data in such a scenario has been approached by Obuchowski[1] and, based on her ideas, a Bayesian technique to estimate the ROC area is developed.

In order to compare modalities and/or readers in multimodality and multi-reader studies, special techniques are required. Lastly, sample size estimation to test hypotheses about diagnostic accuracies are explained and many examples given to elucidate the Bayesian approach.

5.2 Study Design

The elements of good study design for clinical trials of diagnostic tests are explained in the context of the submission of a protocol at MDACC. The Department of Biostatistics and Applied Mathematics first reviews all protocols, which are essentially of two types, those that originate locally here at the institution and those submitted by pharmacutical or medical device companies. For the latter, the protocol is critiqued and reviewed by a statistician in the department. For those studies originating within the institution, a biostatistician would assist the investigator with the design of the study, but the protocol would be reviewed by a different person and presented to the department for approval. The protocol is reviewed by the department and, if necessary, revised according to the suggestions recommended by the departmental consensus. The principal investigator (PI) then revises the protocol, often with the assistance of the statistician.

5.2.1 The Protocol

There are many types of protocols submitted; however, only those dealing mainly with diagnostic tests are considered here. Of course, diagnostic procedures are usually a part of all clinical trials and these will be described in later chapters. Briefly, the protocol outline is:

1. Objectives
2. Background
3. Patient and reader selection
4. Study plan
5. Number of patients
6. Statistical design and analysis
7. References

5.2.2 Objectives

The study's primary and secondary aims are given in the first section of the protocol. The study design is illustrated by a protocol with two nuclear medicine procedures: one using an iodine radionuclide with single photon emission computed tomography (SPECT) (Iodine-123 MIBG (metaiodobenzylguanidine) SPECT) and the other with thallium (Ti- 201 SPECT) that will be used to measure the amount of damage (e.g., scarring of the cardiac wall and nerve damage) to the heart caused by radio therapy to the chest. The main objective is to determine the association between the delivered dose to the target lesion and the nerve damage caused by radiotherapy to the chest. It is an important study because little work in this area has been done.

5.2.3 Background

The recent relevant literature on previous studies should be cited in the Background section of the protocol. It is a very important component because it gives the rationale for doing the study and it often provides information that is essential for sample size estimation. The background information is often a source of preliminary information, which will be employed as prior information for the Bayesian analysis. In the nuclear medicine example, there is a great deal of information on cardiac morbidity and mortality from radiotherapy, but very little on diagnostic imaging procedures that assess the amount of innervation damage. There are only two references citing studies using I-123 MIBG SPECT to assess nerve damage to the heart.

5.2.4 Patient and Reader Selection

The Patient and Reader Selection component provides the inclusion (those who can be admitted) criteria and the ineligibility (those who cannot be admitted) criteria. Generally speaking, those to be included are diseased, but not too diseased to be admitted, while those that are too sick will be excluded. In diagnostic studies when several readers are involved to interpret the diagnostic information, the relationship between how the patients are selected and how the readers are selected must be described. For example, in a traditional selection with two imaging modalities, the same readers will be used to interpret both images and the same patients will be imaged by the two modalities. There are many variations to this scenario, including unpaired patient–unpaired readers, where there are two sets of patients, one for image A and the other for image B, and there are two distinct sets of readers, one for image A and one for image B. Also, there are paired patient and unpaired reader selection plans, etc. For additional selection plans, see Zhou et al.[2], Chap. 3.

If the readers are to interpret two images, is the order randomized to eliminate order bias, and how is a final determination of image interpretation to be handled? How the patients are selected will also affect the sample size estimation, and it could affect any future analysis. For example, the analysis for comparing image accuracy in a paired patient design would be different than that for an unpaired patient selection. If one set of patients is selected at random from a diseased population and the other set selected from a nondiseased population, is this a randomized trial?

Patient and reader selection designs often depend on the type of trial. When developing a new imaging modality, the test should pass three Phases: I, II, and III. The different phases are for different objectives of test accuracy and are as follows: the relation (i.e., paired or unpaired) between patients and the diagnostic modalities and the relation between the readers and modalities should be described in the protocol. The Phase I, II, and III trials for imaging devices were described in a previous chapter, and one is referred to Bogaert et al.[3] for an example of a Phase I developmental trial involving MRI angiography. For an example of a Phase II trial, see Theate et al.[4] and finally for a Phase III trial, see Beam et al.[5] who investigated the interpretation of screening mammograms.

Note that it is important to know the inter-observer variability in these trials because the accuracy of the modality depends not only on the device, but the interpretation of the image via the various readers. Pepe[6] (Chapter 8) gives more detail in the description of developmental trials, and Zhou et al.[2] provide the analysis for studies with multiple readers and multiple modalities for trials of device development.

For the nuclear medicine trial, which is used to motivate the steps involved in the design of a protocol, the paired patients are imaged by both procedures; however, the two modalities will not be compared because they are measuring different things. The iodine radionuclide test is measuring nerve damage to the heart, while the thallium stress test is measuring cardiac perfusion variables, like wall scaring and left ventricular ejection fraction, which are other indicators of cardiac damage.

5.2.5 Study Plan

For this section of the protocol, the details of how the diagnostic tests are to be implemented are spelled out.

Returning to the trial being designed, the study plan is as follows. The sympathetic nervous system of the heart will be imaged using I-123 MIBG, while at the same time performing an exercise stress test using thallium-201 (Tl-201). The patients will be imaged prior to initiation of radiation therapy and at 6 to 12 months after completion of radiation therapy. Stress myocardial perfusion imaging is a standard of care test of baseline evaluation of myocardial perfusion and possible radiation-induced coronary artery disease after radiation therapy of tumors close to the heart. Presently at MDACC, stress myocardial perfusion is performed using the dual isotope method where the patient is injected with thallium-201 for the resting part of the study and, immediately after rest, the patient is injected with technetium-99m (Tc-99m) tetrofosmin at peak stress and imaging is repeated for the stress part of the study.

Next, is the plan to image the patient. This includes details of administering the first radio pharmaceutical I-123 MIBG, including the dose injected intravenously (IV) and how the resulting radioactivity is to be imaged by the gamma camera, in this case SPECT. This is followed by a description of administering the thallium exercise stress test for cardiac perfusion. The patient is imaged with both nuclear medicine procedures before and after radiotherapy. There are two types of cardiac damage variables, those for nerve damage and those measuring scaring of the heart wall and left ventricular ejection fraction, a measure of cardiac output. If radiotherapy is damaging the heart, one would expect to observe it by comparing the post-therapy measurements of heart damage to the corresponding pretherapy values.

Lastly, the image processing details are described. For the cardiac damage study, standard filtered back projection techniques to obtain SPECT images will be employed for both imaging modalities. In order to obtain wall motion images and ejection fraction values, gated motion images are required, thus cardiac motion will not affect the image quality. In order to detect nerve damage, the uptake of norepinephrine can be estimated with the I-123 MIBG SPECT procedure. This illustrates the ability of a nuclear procedure to measure metabolic processes.

5.2.6 Number of Patients

The total number of patients and the monthly accrual rate is described. For multi-institutional trials, the rates for each institution are provided. The total sample size is justified in the power analysis of the statistics section. A maximum of 40 patients accrued at 2 to 3 per month should be sufficient for the cardiac damage protocol.

5.2.7 Statistical Design and Analysis

The statistical section should provide a detailed power analysis that outlines the justification for the sample size. The power analysis should show how the results of previously related studies are used to predict the results of the planned study. It should also provide a brief description of the design of the study, including how the readers and patients interface (i.e., paired with the modalities) with the diagnostic tests. The Phase (I, II, or III) of the study should be identified as well as an outline of how the study results will be analyzed.

For the planning of the Phase I nuclear medicine protocol, the power analysis is as follows: the sample size will be based on the expected association between nerve damage measured by uptake of norepinephrine (as determined by I-123 MIBG) and the dose of radiotherapy (RT) administered to the target lesion measured in Gy (gray unit for absorbed dose of radiation).

If RT is damaging cardiac innervation, one would expect the mean uptake ratio to be 2.5 before RT with a range from 1.5 to 3.5; while after therapy, one would expect the average uptake ratio of norepinephrine to be 1.5 with a range from .5 to 2.5. Assuming a correlation of .5 between pre- and post-therapy for the uptake values of norepinephrine, the standard deviation of the difference is .5.

The independent variable for the association is the RT delivered dose, which will have a range of 40 to 60 Gy, with a average dose of 50 Gy and a standard deviation of 5 Gy. The dose is expected to have an effect on the cardiac nerve damage. When the delivered dose is 40 Gy, it is reasonable to expect an average uptake in the difference to be 0, while if the delivered dose is 60 Gy, it is reasonable to expect the difference in the post minus preuptake values to average 1. Assuming a linear regression between the difference in the uptake values as the dependent variable and the administered dose as the independent variable, the regression line will be approximately

$$Y = .05X - 2$$

where X is the delivered dose in Gy, and Y is the difference in the post minus preRT uptake values. The null hypothesis is that the slope of the regression is zero vs. the alternative hypothesis that the slope is positive. Assuming under the alternative, the slope is .05, the power of the test with an alpha = .05 is .68, .86, and .94 corresponding to sample sizes 20, 30, and 40, respectively. It appears reasonable that 30 patients will show a strong association between damage to the nerves of the heart and the delivered dose to the target lesion.

The power analysis describes what to expect in regard to the nerve damage to the heart in terms of the uptake ratios of norepinephrine, measured before and after radiotherapy. The hypothetical association between the nerve damage and the dose delivered to the target lesion is given by the above regression equation. The power was computed with a standard software package NCSS®, and suggests 30 patients as a reasonable number to detect the desired association. This is somewhat hypothetical in a sense, but is based on previous studies of heart damage caused by radiotherapy to lesions that are close to the heart. The power analysis could just as well be done from a Bayesian perspective (see Broemeling[7] for the Bayesian analysis of a linear regression model).

Note, the power analysis is based on just two of the many endpoints that could have been used. There are many ways to measure cardiac nerve damage and many to measure other damage to the heart, such as left ventricle ejection fraction and scarring to the heart wall. The power analysis should be brief, but at the same time informative, so that other statisticians can review the work.

5.2.8 References

I think of this as the most important section of the protocol because the study is only fit to be run if previous studies show a need. Also, to the statistician, the results from previous studies are invaluable for the power analysis.

5.3 Bayesian Methods for Test Accuracy: Binary and Ordinal Data

5.3.1 Introduction

This section will introduce Bayesian techniques to estimate and test hypotheses concerning the basic measures of test accuracy. The measures of test accuracy are (1) classification probabilities, (2) predictive measures, and (3) diagnostic likelihood ratios. The classification probabilities are the false positive fraction (FPF) and true positive fraction (TPF), while there are two predictive values: the positive predictive value (PPV) and the negative predictive value (NPV). Lastly, there are two diagnostic likelihood ratios, the positive diagnositc likelihood ratio (PDLR) and the negative diagnositc likelihood ratio (NDLR). These measures will be defined in the next section in the context of a cohort study. Thus, there is a random sample of size n selected from the target population and a gold standard, therefore, each patient is classified into four categories in Table 5.1.

TABLE 5.1

Classification Table

Test	$D = 0$	$D = 1$
X = 0	(n_{00}, θ_{00})	(n_{01}, θ_{01})
X = 1	(n_{10}, θ_{10})	(n_{11}, θ_{11})

The n_{ij} are the number of subjects with test score i = 0 or 1 and disease status j = 0 or 1, while θ_{ij} is the corresponding probability.

5.3.2 Classification Probabilities

The basic measures of test accuracy are the TPF (sensitivity) and the FPF (1–specificity) where,

$$\text{TPF}\ (\theta) = \theta_{11}/(\theta_{11} + \theta_{01}) = P(X = 1/D = 1), \tag{5.1}$$

and

$$\text{FPR}\ (\theta) = \theta_{10}/(\theta_{00} + \theta_{10}) = P(X = 1/\text{D} = 0). \tag{5.2}$$

It is important to know that the TPF and FPF are unknown parameters and are functions of θ. The Bayesian analysis determines the posterior distribution of these quantities from which the parameters are estimated and certain tests of hypotheses performed. Assume the prior information is based on a previous study, with results given in Table 5.2

TABLE 5.2

Classification Table of Prior Information

Test	$D = 0$	$D = 1$
$X = 0$	(m_{00}, θ_{00})	(m_{01}, θ_{01})
$X = 1$	(m_{10}, θ_{10})	(m_{11}, θ_{11})

where m subjects have been classified in the same way as those in Table 5.1. The density based on prior information is

$$\xi(\theta) \propto \theta_{00}^{m_{00}} \theta_{01}^{m_{01}} \theta_{10}^{m_{10}} \theta_{11}^{m_{11}}, \tag{5.3}$$

thus, the likelihood function for $\theta = (\theta_{00}, \theta_{01}, \theta_{10}, \theta_{11})$ is

$$L(\theta / n) \propto \theta_{00}^{n_{00}} \theta_{01}^{n_{01}} \theta_{10}^{n_{10}} \theta_{11}^{n_{11}}, \tag{5.4}$$

and the posterior distribution is Dirichlet,

$$\theta/(n, m) \sim Dir\ (n_{00} + m_{00} + 1, n_{01} + m_{01} + 1, n_{10} + m_{10} + 1, n_{11} + m_{11} + 1).$$

If there is no prior information, the m_{ij} are zero, and one, in effect, is assuming a uniform prior distribution for θ.

Direct sampling from the Dirichlet distribution, using Minitab®, will determine the posterior distribution of these classification probabilities. As an example, consider the Coronary Artery Surgery Study (CASS) example examined by Pepe[6] and based on the study by Weiner et al.[7] This is a cohort study of 1465 subjects, where each is classified as to disease status (coronary artery disease (CAD) via an angiogram) and a diagnostic test, the exercise stress test (EST), which is a nuclear medicine procedure (Table 5.3). (See Chapter 2, Section 2.2 for a brief description of nuclear medicine imaging.)

The TPF and FPF are estimated by sampling from their posterior distributions. Since the joint posterior distribution of the parameters is Dirichlet, 1000 samples are generated from their distribution, resulting in four columns of the Minitab worksheet. There is one column for each Dirichlet parameter. The 1000 FPF and TPF values are transformed from the four columns according to Equation (5.1) and Equation (5.2), which give 1000 samples from their

TABLE 5.3

Exercise Stress Test and Heart Disease

EST	$D = 0$	$D = 1$
$X = 0$	327	208
$X = 1$	115	818

TABLE 5.4

Posterior Distribution of TPF and FPF

Parameter	Mean	STD	Median	97. 5% CI
TPF(θ)	.753	.176	.796	(.224, .972)
FPF(θ)	.311	.206	.271	(.024, .803)

posterior distributions. The properties of the posterior distributions are calculated and shown in Table 5.4

A plot of the 1000 values sampled from the joint posterior distribution of (FPF, TPF) is presented in Figure 5.1, along with the histograms of the two marginal posterior distributions.

How does one determine a joint credible region for (TPF, FPF)? Consider the rectangular region (.224, .972) × (.024, .803) for the two parameters, then what is the posterior probability that (TPF, FPF) ∈ (.224, .972) × (.024, .803)? This can be computed from Minitab by creating a column labeled "joint" from the worksheet by the command: "joint'" = (.224 < = 'tpf') and ('tpf' < = .972) and (.024 < = 'fpf') and ('fpf' < = .803). Thus generating 1000 binary values for the "joint" column, with a 0 when the (TPF, FPF) pair is not

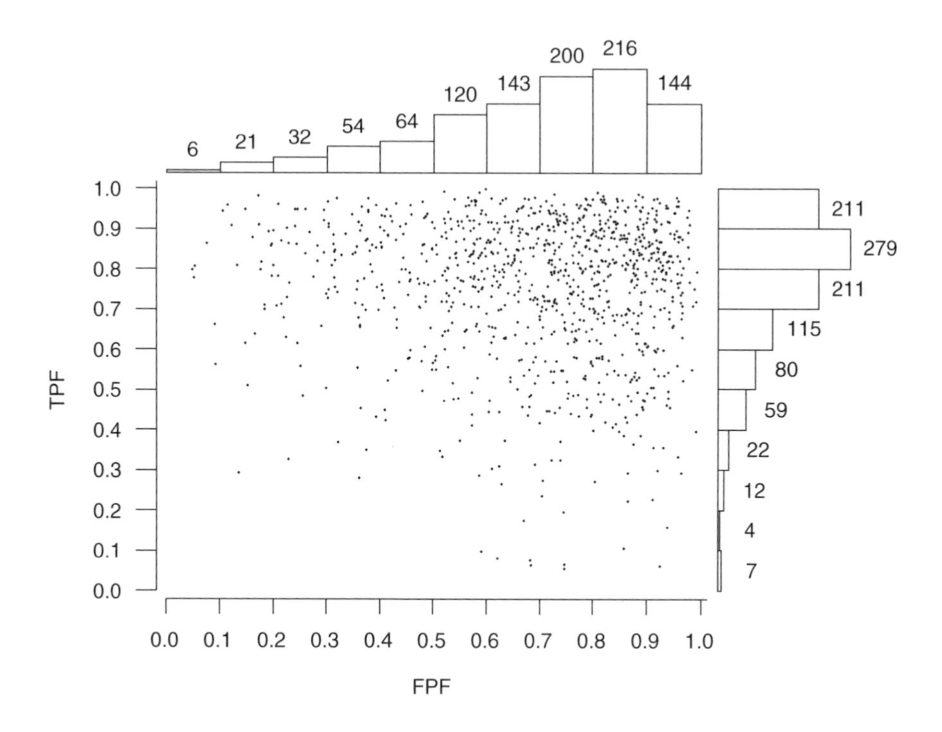

FIGURE 5.1
TPF vs. FPF.

included in the region and with a 1 when it is. Now compute the mean of the "joint" column to give the posterior probability, namely

$$P\{(\text{TPF}, \text{FPF}/\text{data}) \in (.224, .972) \times (.024, .803)\} = .962, \tag{5.5}$$

therefore, the credible region has a posterior content of 96.2% .

Consider a test of the hypothesis H: TPF < FPF vs. A: TPF ≥ FPF. If the posterior probability of the alternative hypothesis is reasonably large, then the null would be rejected in favor of the alternative, but, in fact

$$P(\text{TPF} \geq \text{FPF} / \text{data}) = .586(.492), \tag{5.6}$$

where .492 is the standard deviation. Such a test is important in comparing the sensitivity of the test to its specificity.

5.3.3 Predictive Values

The second set of measures of test accuracy is the positive predictive value (PPV) and the negative predictive value (NPV), defined as follows:

$$\text{PPV}(\theta) = \theta_{11}/(\theta_{01} + \theta_{11}) = P(D = 1/X = 1) \tag{5.7}$$

and

$$\text{NPV}(\theta) = \theta_{00}/(\theta_{00} + \theta_{01}) = P(D = 0/X = 0). \tag{5.8}$$

Since these two quantities depend on disease incidence, it is important that the patients are selected at random from the target population, so that when estimating the predictive values, the estimated disease incidence is done without bias. Returning to the CASS example, the posterior distributions of the predictive values are provided in Table 5.5. They answer the question of primary interest to the patient — Do I have a disease or don't I?

The PPV distribution is skewed to the left, thus a reasonable estimate of it is .868. Note that a perfect test occurs when PPV = NPV = 1.

TABLE 5.5

Distribution of Predictive Values

Parameter	Mean	STD	Median	95 % CI
PPV(θ)	.827	.150	.868	(.400, .984)
NPV(θ)	.585	.220	.606	(.139, .936)

5.3.4 Diagnostic Likelihood Ratios

The diagnostic likelihood ratios are a third group of test accuracy measures and are

$$\begin{aligned} \text{PDLR}(\theta) &= P(X = 1/D = 1)/P(X = 1/D = 0) \\ &= [\theta_{11}/(\theta_{11} + \theta_{01})]/[\theta_{10}/(\theta_{10} + \theta_{00})] \\ &= \text{TPF}(\theta)/\text{FPF}(\theta), \end{aligned} \tag{5.8}$$

and

$$\begin{aligned} \text{NDLR}(\theta) &= P(X = 0/D = 1)/P(X = 0/D = 0) \\ &= [\theta_{01}/(\theta_{11} + \theta_{01})]/[\theta_{00}/(\theta_{10} + \theta_{00})] \\ &= \text{FNF}(\theta)/\text{TNF}(\theta) \end{aligned} \tag{5.9}$$

With regard to the PDLR, the more accurate the diagnostic test becomes, the numerator (TPF) tends to become larger and the denominator (FPF) tends to become smaller, but for the NDLR, the opposite is true, the numerator (FNF) tends to become smaller and the denominator (TNF) tends to become larger. The range of both is $(0, \infty)$.

For the CASS dataset, the characteristics of the posterior distribution are given in Table 5.6.

The posterior distribution of the PDLR is highly skewed to the right with a mean of 4.78 compared to a median of 2.70, therefore, the mean could give a misleading high value for the accuracy. The median PDLR implies the TPF is 2.7 times larger than the FPF. For additional information about these basic measures of accuracy, Pepe[6] provides a summary.

5.3.5 ROC Curve

Consider the results of mammography given to 60 women of which 30 had the disease (Table 5.7). This is presented in Zhou et al.[2]

The radiologist assigns a score from 1 to 5 to each mammogram, where 1 indicates a normal lesion, 2 a benign, 3 a lesion that is probably benign, 4 indicates suspicious, and 5 malignant. How would one estimate the accuracy

TABLE 5.6

Distribution of Diagnostic Likelihood Ratios

Parameter	Mean	STD	Median	95 5% CI
PDLR(θ)	4.780	7.310	2.707	(.726, 20.92)
NDLR(θ)	.424	.466	.3045	(.039, 1.45)

TABLE 5.7

Mammogram Test Results

Status	Normal (1)	Benign (2)	Probably Benign (3)	Suspicious (4)	Malignant (5)	Total
Cancer	1	0	6	11	12	30
No Cancer	9	2	11	8	0	30

for mammography from this information? When the test results are binary, the observed TPF and FPF are calculated, but here there are 5 possible results for each image. The scores could be converted to binary by designating 4 as the threshold, then scores 1 to 3 are negative and 4 to 5 are positive test results. Then estimate the TPF as tpf = 23/30 and the specificity (1 – FPF) as (1 – fpf) = 21/30. Another approach would be to use each test result as a threshold and calculate the tpf and fpf (depicted in Table 5.8).

Of the 30 diseased, 30 had a score of at least 1, while 23 had a score of at least 4. On the other hand, of the 30 without cancer, 30 had a score of at least 1, and 8 had a score of at least 4, etc. Figure 5.2 is a plot of the observed true and false positive values of Table 5.8. What does this graph tell us about the accuracy of mammography?

The area under the ROC gives the intrinsic accuracy of a diagnostic test and can be interpreted in several ways (see Zhou et al.[2]): either as the average sensitivity for all values of specificity, or the average specificity for all values of sensitivity, or as the probability that the diagnostic score of a diseased patient is more of an indication of disease than the score of a patient without the disease or condition. The problem is in determining the area under the curve. For the graph in Figure 5.2, there are five points corresponding to the five threshold values. If the diagnostic score can be considered continuous (e.g., the coronary artery calcium score), then the curve through the points becomes more discernible and the area easier to determine.

In the case of discrete data, the area under the curve as determined by a linear interpolation of the points on the graph (including (0,0) and (1,1)) have the following interpretation:

$$AUC = P(Y > X) + (1/2)P(Y = X). \tag{5.10}$$

See Pepe[6] where it is assumed that one patient is selected at random from the population of diseased patients, with a diagnostic score of Y,

TABLE 5.8

TPF vs. FPF for Mammography Test Results

Status	Normal (1)	Benign (2)	Probably Benign (3)	Suspicious (4)	Malignant (5)
tpf	30/30 = 1.00	30/30 = 1.00	29/30 = .966	23/30 = .766	12/30 = .400
fpf	30/30 = 1.00	21/30 = .700	19/30 = .633	8/30 = .266	0/30 = 0.000

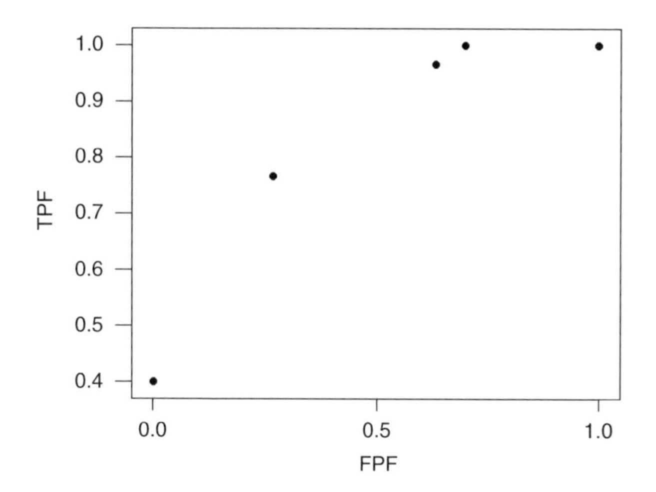

FIGURE 5.2
Empirical ROC graph for mammography.

while another patient, with a score of X, is selected independently from the population of nondiseased patients. Note that the area under the curve (AUC) depends on the parameters of the model. Let us return to the mammography example and estimate the area under the curve via a Bayesian method. The histogram of the posterior distribution of the ROC area is shown in Figure 5.3.

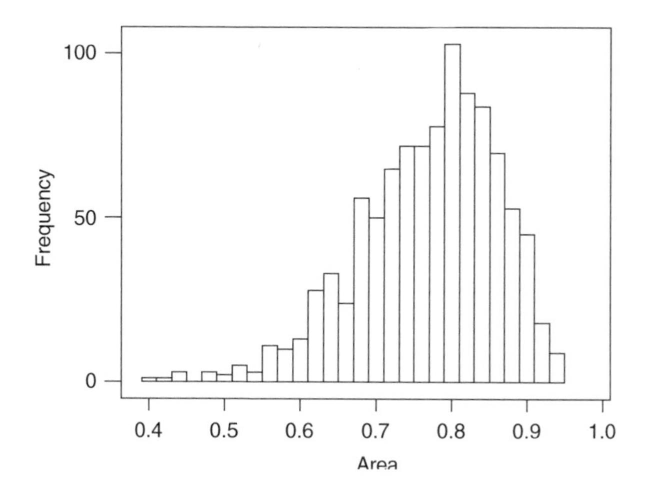

FIGURE 5.3
Posterior distribution of ROC area for mammography.

For the mammography example, the area is defined as

$$AUC\ (\theta, \phi) = P(Y > X/\theta, \phi) + (1/2)P(Y = X/\theta, \phi), \tag{5.11}$$

where Y (= 1, 2, 3, 4, 5) is the diagnostic score for a person with breast cancer and X (=1, 2, 3, 4, 5) for a person without. It can be shown

$$AUC\ (\theta, \phi) = \sum_{i=2}^{i=5} \sum_{j=1}^{j=i-1} \theta_i \phi_j + (1/2) \sum_{i=1}^{i=5} \theta_i \phi_i. \tag{5.12}$$

It is assumed the Y and X are independent, given the parameters, and that

$$P(Y = \mathrm{i}) = \theta_i \quad \text{and} \quad \mathrm{P}(X = j) = \phi_j, \quad i, j = 1,2,3,4,5.$$

AUC is a parameter that depends on θ and ϕ.

Their posterior distributions are $\theta/data \sim Dir\ (2, 17, 12, 13)$ and independent of $\phi/data \sim Dir\ (10, 3, 12, 9, 1)$, assuming a uniform prior for the parameters (see Table 5.7).

Samples from the posterior distribution of the AUC are generated by sampling from the posterior distributions of θ and ϕ. This was done with Minitab, where 5 columns of the worksheet were used to generate 1000 samples from the Dirichlet posterior distribution of θ, and 5 columns to generate 1000 samples from the posterior distribution of ϕ. Consequently, using Formula (5.12), 1000 values are computed from the posterior distribution of AUC. The mean and median of the posterior distribution of AUC are .768 and .782, respectively; the standard deviation is .091 and a 95% credible interval (.560, .910). The skewness to the left produces a "wide" interval estimate of the ROC area. This value is to be compared to the value found by Zhou et al.[2]

Lastly, the mammography example is concluded with a test for the usefulness of the procedure. Obviously, a perfect test has an ROC area of 1, and a useless test area of .5. Thus, consider a Bayesian test of H: AUC < .5 vs. the alternative A: AUC ≥ .5. How is this performed with Minitab? From the worksheet, create a column with the command area > .5, which will generate 1000 binary values: 0 when the condition is not satisfied and 1 when it is. The mean of this column is the probability of the alternative hypothesis and

$$P(AUC(\theta, \phi) \geq .5/\mathrm{data}) = .991.$$

Therefore, by this criterion, mammography is a useful procedure.

5.4 Bayesian Methods for Test Accuracy: Quantitative Variables

5.4.1 Introduction

The methods introduced previously for discrete diagnostic tests apply to quantitative variables as well. The basic measures of test accuracy, including classification probabilities, predictive measures, and diagnostic likelihood ratios, all apply to continuous variables, such as blood glucose levels to diagnose diabetes, the levels of glucose metabolism in nuclear medicine procedures, and the PSA (prostate specific antigen) levels to help diagnose prostate cancer. Other quantitative variables to be considered in this book are coronary artery calcium (CAC) levels in coronary heart disease, and standardized uptake levels to assess metastasis to the spinal column.

In clinical practice, quantitative variables are often dichotomized. For example, CAC levels in excess of 400, PSA levels in excess of 4 ng/ml, and blood glucose levels in excess of 126 mg/dL are standard threshold values. Of course, with a threshold value and a gold standard, the diagnostic accuracy can be estimated with the Bayesian methods previously introduced. In this section, methods for choosing a threshold value are explained in the context of a cost benefit analysis.

The primary focus on test accuracy will be the area under the ROC curve. Its mathematical properties will be outlined and Bayesian methods of estimating the area explained.

5.4.2 The Spokane Heart Study

The Spokane Heart Study was conducted at Washington State University and the CT imaging was implemented at the Shields Coronary Artery Center in Spokane. Over a period of 10 years there were nearly 4400 patient visits, where cardiologist referred the majority of the patients. Thus, the relevant population was community based and a comprehensive history was taken of each patient's symptoms. These patients had confirmed coronary artery disease or were at high risk for the disease.

At the time, the use of CAC to assist in the diagnosis and patient management was not an accepted standard procedure; however, since then it is gradually being accepted. There are several experimental studies that involve a CT (computed tomography) determination of the CAC in the coronary arteries. Measurements of CAC were made with the Imatron C-100 Ultrafast CT Scanner. The description of the Spokane study is given in Mielke et al.[9] The CAC score is a positive score and is the sum of several CAC scores corresponding to the various coronary arteries and gives a measure of the amount of plaque burden.

Rumberger et al.[10] developed a risk index for CAD by categorizing the CAC scores as follows:

- A value of 1 is a CAC score of zero and indicates very low risk.
- A value of 2 is assigned for CAC scores between 1 and 10 and represents low risk of disease.
- CAC scores between 11 and 100 indicated a moderate risk and are assigned a value of 3.
- A value of 4 is assigned to scores between 101 and 400 for high risk.
- A very high risk has a value of 5 for CAC scores greater than 400.

With the occurrence of infarction as a gold standard, the 130 patients who had an infarct were assigned the following risk scores:

Very low risk: 12

Low risk: 6

Moderate risk: 27

High risk: 40

Very high risk: 45

As for the 4263 patients who did not experience an infarct, they were assigned to the following risk categories.

Very low risk: 1818

Low risk: 527

Moderate risk: 814

High risk: 648

Very high risk: 454

Assuming a uniform prior distribution for the parameters, the posterior distribution of $\theta = (\theta_1, \theta_2, \theta_3, \theta_4, \theta_5)$ is Dirichlet (13, 7, 28, 41, 46), where θ_1 is the probability a diseased patient has a low risk of disease, etc., and in a similar fashion, the posterior distribution of $\phi = (\phi_1, \phi_2, \phi_3, \phi_4, \phi_5)$ is Dirichlet (1819, 528, 815, 649, 455), where ϕ_5 is the probability a patient without an infarct has a very high risk of disease. If high risk is the threshold, it can be shown that the TPF (θ) has a Beta distribution with mean .626, median .639, and standard deviation .150. On the hand, the FPF (ϕ) has a Beta posterior distribution with mean .272, median .251, and standard deviation .133.

5.4.3 ROC Area

The area under the ROC curve gives an intrinsic value to the accuracy of a diagnostic test and has a long history beginning in signal detection theory. See Egan[11] for the early use of the ROC curve in signal detection theory. Also, the books by Pepe[6] and Zhou et al.[2] provide the history as well as the latest statistical methods (non Bayesian) for using ROC curves in diagnostic medicine. The ROC area is generally accepted as the way to measure diagnostic accuracy in radiology.

Let X be a quantitative variable and r a threshold value, and consider the test positive when $X \geq r$, otherwise negative, then the ROC curve is the set of all points

$$\begin{aligned} \text{ROC}(.) &= \{ [\text{FPF}(r), \text{TPF}(r)], r \text{ any real number}\} \\ &= \{[t, \text{ROC}(t)], t \in (0, 1)\}, \end{aligned} \tag{5.13}$$

where t = FPF(r), that is, r is the threshold corresponding to t. As r becomes large, FPF(r) and TPF(r) tend to zero, while if r becomes small, FPF(r) and TPF(r) tend to 1, thus the ROC curve passes through (0,0) and (1,1). If the area under the curve is 1, the test is discriminating perfectly between the diseased and nondiseased groups, while if the area is .5, the test cannot discriminate between the two groups.

Chapter 4 of Pepe presents several useful properties of the ROC curve: (1) the invariance of the ROC curve under monotone increasing transformations of X, (2) interpreting the ROC area for continuous variables as AUC = $P(X > Y)$, and (3) a formula for the AUC area when X is normally distributed.

The Bayesian approach to estimating the ROC area is based on AUC = $\Phi [a/\sqrt{1+b^2}]$, where X is normally distributed, $a = (\mu_D - \mu_{\bar{D}})/\sigma_D$, and $b = \sigma_D/\sigma_{\bar{D}}$. The mean and standard deviation of the X for the diseased population are μ_D and σ_D, respectively, while $\mu_{\bar{D}}$ and $\sigma_{\bar{D}}$ are the mean and standard deviation of X for the nondiseased. Φ is the cumulative distribution function of the standard normal distribution. This formula is cited by many authors; however, Pepe presents an excellent discussion of its use.

Note the ROC area AUC depends on the unknown parameters of the model. Bayesian methods for estimating the ROC area will be illustrated by referring to an example found in Zhou et al., which is based on the study by Hans et al.[12] The data are given in Table 4.12 of Zhou and refer to the use of CK-BB, an enzyme in the spinal fluid collected within 24 hours of injury, to predict the outcome of severe trauma.

The WinBUGS® statements below are a modification of those presented by O'Malley et al.[13] The program is based on the binormal assumption, where the diagnostic variable X has a normal distribution for both populations. The model is a linear regression model with three regression coefficients: a constant, the group effect, and an effect for age. If the covariable is not to be included, delete the third regression coefficient beta 3. The first level parameters are the μs and precisions of the observations (the CK-BB levels, one for each patient) where each patient has a mean expressed as a linear regression on the group effect and the age effect. The regression coefficients are second-level parameters and given uninformative normal distributions, while the two precision parameters are given noninformative gamma distributions.

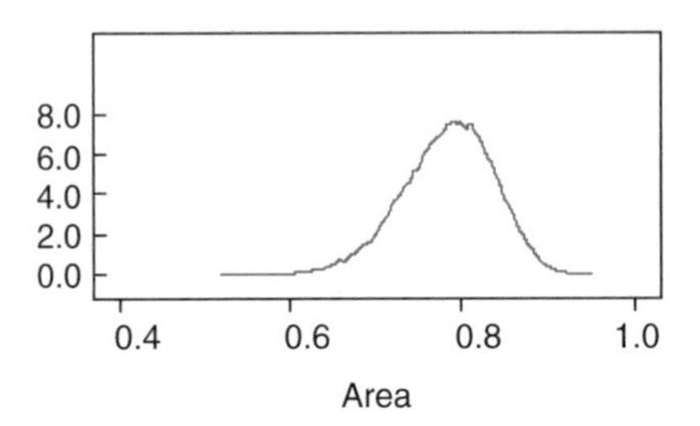

FIGURE 5.4
AUC area CB-KK.

There are two list statements, the first of which consists of three vectors for the data. The y vector lists the CK-BB values, the vector d is a group identification vector, and the third vector age lists the age of each patient. The second list statement specifies the initial values for the Monte Carlo Markov Chain (MCMC) algorithm. The vector beta lists the initial values for the regression coefficients, and the vector precy, the initial values for the two precision parameters.

There are 60 patients, 19 who do not have severe trauma. The primary parameters of the AUC are a and b. The initial run is made without the covariable. The characteristics of the posterior AUC area are: mean = .783, median = .787, std = .052, a 95% credible interval of (.670, .875), and the plot of the posterior distribution for the area in Figure 5.4. The refreshing sequence length is 500 samples, and 75,000 samples were generated from the posterior distribution of AUC, with an MC error of .0002103. See Table 5.9 for additional results of the posterior analysis. These results are comparable to Zhou et al.[2], which gave an area of .790, based on the original observations and the property (4) above. They also estimated the area as .818 with the logs of the observations.

TABLE 5.9
Posterior Distribution of AUC

Parameter	Mean	STD	Lower 21/2	Median	Upper 21/2
a	.823	.190	.452	.822	1.201
b	.253	.053	.167	.247	.376
auc	.783	.052	.670	.787	.875

```
model
{
# likelihood function
for(i in 1:N) {

y[i]~ dnorm(mu[i],precy[d[i]+1]);
```

```
#   yt[i] <- log(y[i]); # logarithmic transformation
mu[i] <- beta[1] + beta[2]*d[i] + beta[3]*age[i] ;
}
# prior distributions  noninformative prior; similarly
for informative priors
for(i in 1:P) {
beta[i] ~ dnorm(0, 0.000001);
}
for(i in 1:K) {
precy[i]~dgamma(0.001, 0.001);
vary[i] <- 1.0/precy[i];}
# calculates area under the curve
a <- beta[2]/sqrt(vary[2]); # ROC curve parameters
la2 <- vary[1]/vary[2];
auc <- phi(a/sqrt(1+la2)
b<- sqrt(la2)
fpf<- phi((a*b-sqrt(a*a+2*(1-b*b)*log(ka/b))/(1-b*b)))
tpf<- phi((a - b*sqrt(a*a+(1-b*b)*log(ka/b))/(1-
b*b)));}
list (K=2, P=3, N=60,
y=c(140,1087,230,183,1256,700,16,800,253,740,126,153,
283,90,303,193,76,1370,543,913,230,463,60,509,576,671
,80,490,156,356,350,323,1560,120,216,443,523,76,303,3
53,206,136,286,281,23,200,146,220,96,100,60,17,27,126
,100,253,70,40,6,46),
d=c(1,1,1,1,1,1,1,1,1,1,1,1,1,1,1,1,1,1,1,1,1,1,1,1,1
,1,1,1,1,1,1,1,1,1,1,1,1,1,1,1,0,0,0,0,0,0,0,0,0,0,
0,0,0,0,0,0,0,0,0),
age=c(4,7,8,11,15,16,16,16,17,18,18,18,19,19,19,19,20
,20,20,20,20,21,22,23,23,24,29,29,29,30,40,41,45,45,5
0,51,56,59,61,61,62,6,6,7,8,8,10,11,12,12,16,17,18,18
,19,24,28,35,38,46))
list(beta=c(0,0,0),precy=c(1,1))
```

5.4.4 Definition of the ROC Curve

The ROC curve is defined by Equation (5.13) and under the assumption of binormality has the representation

$$[t, 1 - \Phi\,(bZ_t - a)]\ \mathrm{t} \in (0, 1), \tag{5.14}$$

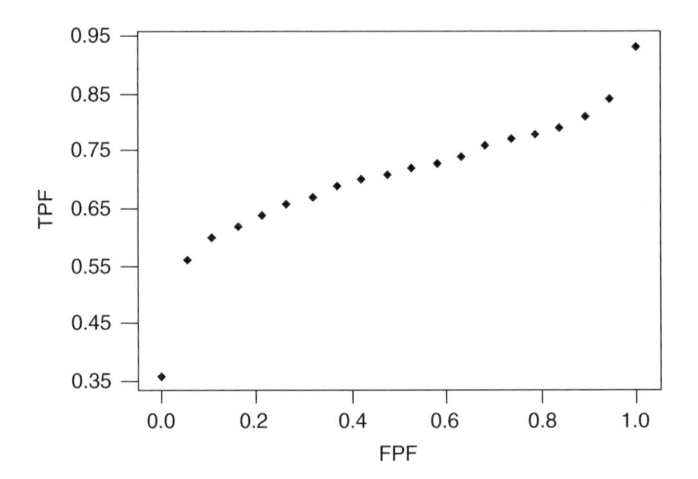

FIGURE 5.5
Binormal ROC curve head trauma study.

where t is the FPF, $t = 1 - \Phi(Z_t)$, thus Z_t is the upper t percentage point of the standard normal distribution. Note that a and b are unknown parameters and have a posterior distribution. Therefore, what should be used for the values of a and b in Equation (5.14) when plotting the curve?

If the posterior medians of a and b are used (see Table 5.9), the graph for the ROC curve is given in Figure 5.5.

5.4.5 Choice of Optimal Threshold Value

Cost considerations are often used to select a threshold value for a diagnostic test. For example, Zhou et al.[2] base the choice of an optimal cutoff value on minimizing the total cost

$$C = \text{TPF}\, p\, (C_{tp} - C_{fn}) + \text{FPF}(1 - p)\, (C_{fp} - C_{tn}) + C_0 + pC_{fn} + (1 - p)C_{tn},$$

where p is the disease incidence, C_0 is the cost of performing the test, while C_{tp}, C_{fn}, C_{fp} and C_{tn} are the costs of a true positive, false negative, false positive, and true negative, respectively. When this expression is differentiated with respect to FPF, the slope to the curve at the optimal point is

$$\kappa = (1-p)R/p,$$

where (5.15)

$$R = (C_{tn} - C_{fp})/(C_{tp} - C_{fn}).$$

TABLE 5.10

Posterior Distribution Coordinates of Optimal Point κ = .5

Coordinates	Mean	STD	Lower $2^1/_2$	Median	Upper $2^1/_2$
TPF	.692	.051	.584	.694	.786
FPF	.096	.028	.056	.094	.167

Assuming binormality, Somoza and Mossman[14] have shown that the optimal point is (FPF, TPF) where

$$FPF(a,b) = \phi\left\{[ab - \sqrt{a^2 + 2(1-b^2)\ln(\kappa / b)}] / (1-b^2)\right\}$$

and (5.16)

$$TPF(a,b) = \phi\left\{[a - b\sqrt{a^2 + (1-b^2)\ln(\kappa / b)}] / (1-b^2)\right\}.$$

Treating κ as a constant, the coordinates of the optimal point are functions of the parameters a and b and have posterior distributions. Assuming binormality, Zhou et al. Equation (5.16) of the optimal point for values of κ for $R = .5, 1, 1.5$ and $p = .2, .5, .67$.

The statements corresponding to Equation (5.16) appear in the above worksheet. Generating 75,000 samples from the joint posterior distribution (fpf, tpf) with a refreshing sequence of length 500, the posterior distribution of the coordinates of the optimal point are shown in Table 5.10 for κ = .5 (p = .5 and R = 1). What is the threshold for CB-KK corresponding to the coordinates of the optimal point?

5.5 Clustered Data: Detection and Localization

5.5.1 Introduction

In assessing the area under the receiver operating characteristics (ROC) curve for the accuracy of a diagnostic test, it is imperative to detect and locate multiple abnormalities per image. This approach takes this into account by adopting a statistical model that allows for correlation between the reader scores of several regions of interest (ROI).

The ROI method of partitioning the image is taken. The readers give a score to each ROI in the image and the statistical model takes into account the correlation between the scores of the ROIs (regions of interest) of an image in estimating test accuracy. The test accuracy is given by $P(Y > Z) + (1/2)P(Y = Z)$

where Y is a discrete diagnostic measurement of an affected ROI and Z is the diagnostic measurement of an unaffected ROI. This way of measuring test accuracy is equivalent to the area under the ROC curve. The parameters are the parameters of a multinomial distribution. Based on the multinomial distribution, a Bayesian method of inference is adopted for estimating the test accuracy.

Using a multinomial model for the test results, a Bayesian method based on the predictive distribution of future diagnostic scores is employed to find the test accuracy. By resampling from the posterior distribution of the model parameters, samples from the posterior distribution of test accuracy are also generated. Using these samples, the posterior mean, standard deviation, and credible intervals are calculated in order to estimate the area under the ROC curve. A Bayesian way to estimate test accuracy is easy to perform with standard software packages and has the advantage of employing the efficient inclusion of information from prior related imaging studies.

Obuchowski et al.[1] demonstrate how the ROI method is used to estimate the area under the ROC curve. They conclude that the ROI method appropriately captures the detection and localization of multiple abnormalities and is better suited than the free-response ROC curve method. In the ROI approach, the image is partitioned into clinically relevant, mutually exclusive regions. For example, in mammography, there are five ROIs: upper outer, upper inner, lower outer, lower inner, and retroareolar. The reader assigns a score to each ROI that ranges from 1 to 5 as to the confidence of the presence of an abnormality, thus the reader's ability to find abnormalities and to locate them is easily determined. They continue by presenting a way to take into account the correlation between the scores of the several ROIs of the same image. I will not go into the details of the Obuchowski et al. study, but will adopt their ROI approach as the preferred method of assessing test accuracy when there are many ROIs per image.

5.5.2 Bayesian ROC Curve for Clustered Information

The proposed method is based on the ROI (not on a per patient basis) method and the Bayesian way to make statistical inferences. Suppose that a ROI is selected at random from a group of m affected (based on the gold standard) ROIs and let Y be the ordinal diagnostic measurement observed on that ROI, and let Z be the measurement of an ROI selected at random from the set of n unaffected ROIs. The accuracy of the test is given by the area under the ROC curve and is estimated by

$$P(Y > Z) + P(Y = Z)/2 \tag{5.17}$$

and provides the investigator with the overall accuracy of the diagnostic test.

Suppose Y and Z have possible values 1, 2, 3, 4,..., and r where larger values are more of an indication that the ROI is affected; the study results then can be represented by the following likelihood function for θ and ϕ.

$$L(\theta,\phi/y,z) \propto \prod_{i=1}^{i=r} \theta_i^{Y_i}\phi_i^{Z_i}, \tag{5.18}$$

where $\theta = (\theta_1, \theta_2,\ldots,\theta_r)$ and $\phi = (\phi_1, \phi_2,\ldots,\phi_r)$. The diagnostic measurement of an affected ROI is such that $Y = i$ with probability θ_i.

Similarly, for an unaffected ROI, $Z = i$ with probability ϕ_i where Y_i is the frequency of $Y = i$ and Z_i the frequency that $Z = i$ ($i = 1,2,\ldots,$ r).

Note that this likelihood function is based on the multinomial distribution. We see that $\Sigma_{i=1}^{i=r}(\theta_i + \phi_i) = 1$, $\Sigma_{i=1}^{i=r} Y_i = m$, and $\Sigma_{i=1}^{i=r} Z_i = n$. For a given study, the values of m, n, the Y_i, and the Z_i are known, but the θ_i and ϕ_i are not and must be estimated from the data.

To do this using the Bayesian approach, a prior density for the parameters must be specified. Suppose

$$g(\theta,\phi) \propto \prod_{i=1}^{i=r} \theta_i^{\alpha_i-1}\phi_i^{\beta_i-1}$$

is the prior density, then the posterior density of the model parameters is

$$g(\theta,\phi / y,z) \propto \prod_{i=1}^{i=r} \theta_i^{Y_i+\alpha_i-1}\phi_i^{Z_i+\beta_i-1} \tag{5.19}.$$

The posterior density is that of a Dirichlet distribution and the θ_i and ϕ_i are correlated. Because of the constraint, the correlation between the probabilities of the scores of the affected and unaffected ROIs have been taken into account, an essential requirement for the ROI method of detection and localization.

The posterior distribution of $\theta = (\theta_1,\theta_2,\ldots,\theta_r)$ and $\phi = (\phi_1,\phi_2,\ldots,\phi_r)$ is Dirichlet with parameter $(Y_1 + \alpha_1, Y_2 + \alpha_2,\ldots,Y_r + \alpha_r, Z_1 + \beta_1, Z_2 + \beta_2,\ldots,Z_r + \beta_r)$.

It should be stressed that the prior distribution must be chosen with care. There are essentially two cases to consider: (1) prior information from previous related experiments, and (2) little prior information is available. We will discuss this further when examples are to be illustrated.

If one lets

$$\theta_i^* = \theta_i \Big/ \sum_{i=1}^{i=r} \theta_i, \tag{5.20}$$

then θ_i^* is the probability that $Y = i$ when sampling only from the affected ROIs. Suppose an ROI is selected at random from the population of unaffected

ROIs, then ϕ_i^* is the probability that $Z = i$ where

$$\phi_i^* = \phi_i \Big/ \sum_{i=1}^{i=r} \phi_i. \tag{5.21}$$

How does the probability $Pr(Y > Z) + (1/2)Pr(Y = Z)$ depends on the model parameters? The following gives the number of ways that $Y \geq Z$ and the corresponding probabilities.

1. Y = 1 and Z = 1 with probability $\theta_1^* \phi_1^*$, or
2. $Y = 2$ and $Z = 1$ or 2 with probability $\theta_2^*(\phi_1^* + \phi_2^*)$, or

.

.

.

r. $Y = r$ and $Z = 1$ or 2 or, . . . or r with probability θ_r^*.

In general, the area under the ROC curve is defined as

$$A(\theta, \phi) = \sum_{i=2}^{i=r} \theta_i^* \sum_{j=1}^{j=i-1} \phi_j^* + (1/2) \sum_{i=1}^{i=r} \theta_i^* \phi_i^*. \tag{5.22}$$

Suppose a "large" number M (say, 10,000) samples are generated from the posterior Dirichlet distribution of θ and ϕ, then this provides M samples generated from the posterior distribution of θ^* and ϕ^* via Equation (5.19), Equation (5.20) and Equation (5.21), and also provides M samples from the posterior distributions of $A(\theta, \phi)$ via Equation (5.22). Based on these samples, the posterior mean, median, standard deviation, and 95% credible interval (or other posterior characteristic) are easily computed.

How large is M? One way to choose M is to choose it large enough so that the generated posterior mean of θ_1 agrees (to, say, two decimal places) with its known true value. Since the posterior distribution of θ_1 is Beta, its mean is known, and can be compared to the value computed by resampling.

5.5.3 Clustered Data in Mammography

This method for clustered data is illustrated from an example taken from Zhou et al.[2] and is based on a study of mammography where there are five ROIs: upper outer, upper inner, lower outer, lower inner, and retroareolar for the right breast. The reader assigns a score to each ROI that ranges from 1 to 4 that indicates the degree of malignancy. There are 58 patients and for each a score from 1 to 4 was assigned to each of the five ROIs. As determined by a gold standard, there were 15 abnormal (malignant) ROIs and 275 normal (non-malignant) ROIs. Assuming a uniform prior for the parameters, the joint posterior distribution of $\theta = (\theta_1, \theta_2, \ldots \theta_4)$ and $\phi = (\phi_1, \phi_2, \ldots \phi_4)$ is Dirichlet with parameter

(6, 1, 3, 9, 236, 16, 11, 16), that is to say, among the abnormal ROIs, 5 had a score of 1, none with a score of 2, 2 with a score of 3, and 8 with a score of 4. Among the malignant ROIs, there are 235 with a score of 1, 15 with a score of 2, 10 with a score 3, and 15 with a value of 4. Increasing values of the diagnostic score indicate a larger chance of malignancy. The area under the curve is

$$A(\theta,\phi)=\sum_{i=2}^{i=4}\theta_i^*\sum_{j=1}^{j=i-1}\phi_j^*+(1/2)\sum_{i=1}^{i=4}\theta_i^*\phi_i^*. \tag{5.23}$$

Using Minitab, 1000 values were generated from the Dirichlet (6, 1, 3, 9, 236, 16, 11, 16) posterior distribution of θ and ϕ. Eight columns of generated values were determined where the first four columns were for the theta parameters and the remaining for the phi parameters. The correlation between these are shown in Table 5.11.

Then, 1000 values are computed from the posterior distribution of the $\theta_i^*=\theta_i/\Sigma_{i=1}^{i=4}\theta_i$ and $\phi_i^*=\phi_i/\Sigma_{i=1}^{i=4}\phi_i$, and, lastly, 1000 values from the ROC area (5.23). The histogram of the posterior distribution is given in Figure 5.6.

The characteristics of the posterior distribution are: mean = .759, median = .774, std = .115, and a 95% credible interval (.503, .906). On the other hand, Zhou et al. report an ROC area of .8098 (.0679). Taking into account the skewness of the posterior distribution, the median is comparable to their estimate. The formula (5.23) of the ROC area is based on a linear interpolation of the 6 points, including (0,0) and (1,1), on the empirical ROC graph. Alternatively, suppose the ROC area is based instead on

$$P(Y\geq Z/\text{parameters}) \text{ or, equivalently,}$$

$$A(\theta,\phi)=\sum_{i=2}^{i=4}\theta_i^*\sum_{j=1}^{j=i-1}\phi_j^*+\sum_{i=1}^{i=4}\theta_i^*\phi_i^*,$$

then the ROC area is estimated by: mean = .910, median = .934, std = .076 , and 95% credible interval (.697, .987). The median estimate of the area is .16

TABLE 5.11

Correlations between Normal and Abnormal ROI Parameters Mammography Clustered Data

	θ_1	θ_2	θ_3	θ_4	ϕ_1	ϕ_2	ϕ_3	ϕ_4
θ_2	.309							
θ_3	.387	.268						
θ_4	.237	.297	.331					
ϕ_1	−.543	−.483	−.543	−.593				
ϕ_2	.290	.251	.309	.270	−.670			
ϕ_3	.303	.361	.349	.340	−.675	.280		
ϕ_4	.227	.297	.247	.235	−.700	.235	.307	

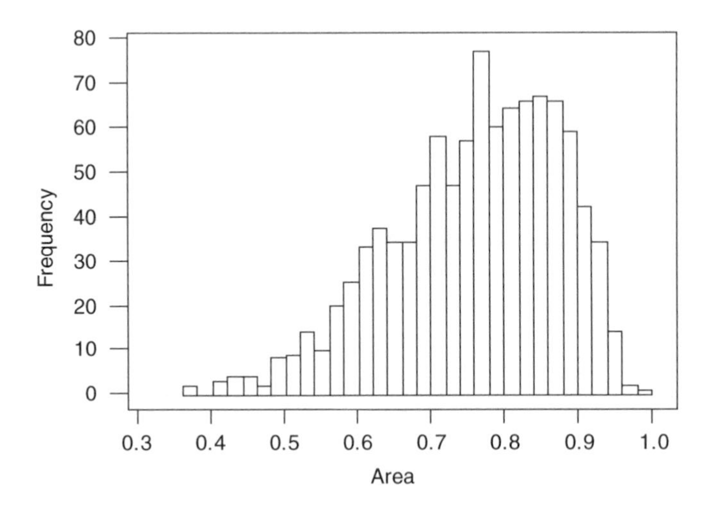

FIGURE 5.6
Posterior distribution ROC area: clustered mammography information.

larger than previously and is .125 larger than that reported by Zhou et al. I would expect the first Bayesian estimate to underestimate the area because it is based on linear interpolation of 4 points on the graph. Also, I would expect the latter Bayesian estimate to overestimate the area because the formula $P(Y \geq Z/\text{parameters})$ is an appropriate estimate when the data are continuous.

5.6 Comparing Accuracy between Modalities

To compare modalities, the CASS dataset is again used where the EST (exercise stress test) and CPH (chest pain history) are used to diagnose coronary artery disease. The example was employed to illustrate the Bayesian estimation of the basic measures of test accuracy (see Section 5.3), including the classification probabilities, diagnostic likelihood ratios, and the predictive probabilities. There are 1465 subjects all of who had an EST and a record of chest pain. This paired study is given in Table 5.12 (see Pepe[6]).

TABLE 5.12A
CASS Study for Diseased Subjects

	CPH		
	0	1	Total
EST			
0	25	183	208
1	29	786	815
Total	54	969	1023

TABLE 5.12B

CASS Study for Nondiseased Subjects

	CPH		
	0	**1**	**Total**
EST			
0	151	176	327
1	46	69	115
Total	197	245	442

The Bayesian analysis will consist of finding the posterior distribution of the sensitivity and specificity of the two modalities and comparing them on the basis of the ratios of the two basic measures. Let θ_{ij} be the probability that a diseased subject has an EST score of i and a record of chest pain j where $i, j = 0, 1$ and where 0 indicates negative outcome and 1 indicates a positive. In a similar manner, let ϕ_{ij} be the corresponding probability for a nondiseased subject.

Assuming a uniform prior distribution for $\theta = (\theta_{00},\theta_{01},\theta_{10},\theta_{11})$ and $\phi = (\phi_{00},\phi_{01},\phi_{10},\phi_{11})$, their joint posterior distribution is Dirichlet with parameter (26, 184, 30, 787; 152, 177, 47, 70). Note that this is a joint posterior distribution of eight parameters. The truncated distribution of θ is the distribution of the

$$\theta_{ij} \Big/ \sum_{i=0}^{i=1}\sum_{j=0}^{j=1}\theta_{ij} = \theta_{ij}^{*}. \tag{5.24}$$

and the truncated distribution of ϕ is the distribution of the

$$\phi_{ij}^{*} = \sum_{i=0}^{i=1}\sum_{j=0}^{j=1}\phi_{ij}. \tag{5.25}$$

The sensitivity (TPF) for EST and CPH are

$$\text{Senest} = \theta_{1.}^{*}. \tag{5.26}$$

and

$$\text{Sencph} = \theta_{.1}^{*} \tag{5.27}$$

respectively, where the dot notation indicates summation of the θ_{ij}^{*} over the missing subscript. In a similar way, the specificity (1 – FPF) for the EST and CPH modalities are

$$\text{Spest} = \phi_{1.}^{*} \tag{5.28}$$

and

$$\text{Spcph} = \phi^*_{.1} \tag{5.29}$$

respectively.

Also, the area under the ROC curve for EST is

$$\text{Aest} = \sum_{i=0}^{i=1} \theta^*_{i.}\phi^*_{i.}/2 + \theta^*_{1.}\phi^*_{0.} \tag{5.30}$$

and for CPH

$$\text{Acph} = \sum_{i=0}^{i=1} \theta^*_{.i}\phi^*_{.i}/2 + \theta^*_{.1}\phi^*_{.0}. \tag{5.31}$$

The posterior distribution for eight multinomial parameters $\theta = (\theta_{00},\theta_{01},\theta_{10},\theta_{11})$ and $\phi = (\phi_{00},\phi_{01},\phi_{10},\phi_{11})$ were determined with Minitab by generating 1000 values in 8 columns of the worksheet. Then the values used for the truncated distributions of the θ^*_{ij} and ϕ^*_{ij} the were computed via (5.24) and (5.25), giving 8 more columns in the worksheet . Additional columns for the various measures of accuracy were computed from the appropriate formulas above. The descriptive statistics for these columns provide the posterior mean, standard deviation, and median. The 95% credible intervals were computed by sorting the 1000 values in ascending order and using the 25th and 975th values as estimates of the lower and upper $2\frac{1}{2}$% points, respectively, of the posterior distribution.

The sensitivity and specificity between the EST and CPH are compared on the basis of a ratio, while the ROC areas between modalities are compared by the difference in the areas. It appears from Table 5.13 that the

TABLE 5.13

Comparison between EST and CPH

Parameter	Mean	Median	STD	Credible Interval
EST Sensitivity	.756	.798	.162	
CPH Sensitivity	.928	.943	.052	
rsen(CPH,EST)	1.316	1.172	.523	.978, 2.51
EST Specificity	.716	.738	.135	
CPH Specificity	.450	.444	.172	
rsp(CPH,EST)	.657	.628	.301	.170, 1.293
ROC Area ETS*	.736	.753	.103	
ROC Area CPH*	.689	.686	.090	
ROC Area ETS**	.932	.948	.058	
ROC Area CPH**	.960	.969	.033	
Difference* ROC Areas	−.047	.047	.131	−.216, .278
Difference** ROC Areas	−.028	−.016	.058	−.172, .059

*Based on the $P(Y > Z/\theta^*, \phi^*) + (1/2)P(Y = Z/\theta^*, \phi^*)$

**Based on $P(Y \geq Z/\theta^*, \phi^*)$.

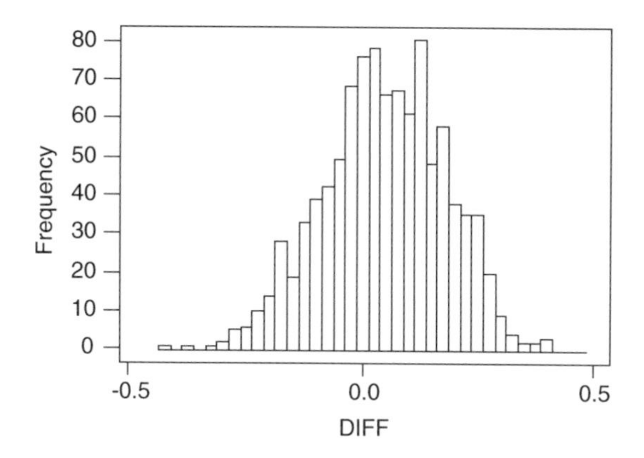

FIGURE 5.7
Posterior distribution histogram of difference in ROC area EST minus CPH.

two modalities are different with regard to sensitivity and specificity, but not with respect to the area under the ROC curve. The histogram of the difference of the ROC area of EST and the ROC area of CPH is given by Figure 5.7.

In order to compare the sensitivities of the two modalities, consider a test of

$$H\text{: rsen(CPH,EST)} < 1 \text{ vs. } A\text{: rsen(CPH,EST)} > 1$$

where

$$\text{rsen(CPH,EST)} = \text{sencph/senets.}$$

It may be shown that the posterior probability of the alternative hypothesis is

$$P(\text{rsen(CPH,EST)} > 1/\text{data}) = .950(.211). \tag{5.32}$$

5.7 Sample Size Determination

5.7.1 Introduction

An important element in designing an experiment is to estimate the sample size that is necessary to accomplish the objectives of the study. As we have seen, the study objectives are specified in the protocol where they are rephrased in statistical language, usually in terms of testing hypotheses. Beginning with discrete diagnostic tests, sample sizes for one test and then for two diagnostic tests are estimated with a Bayesian foundation. Sample sizes for tests concerning hypotheses about the basic measures of accuracy are derived, then these are extended to tests of hypotheses about areas of ROC curves, both for a single diagnostic procedure or for comparing ROC areas between two modalities or readers. The section is concluded with a sample size estimation for continuous diagnostic scores where the binormal assumption is appropriate.

5.7.2 Discrete Diagnostic Scores

Assuming discrete diagnostic scores, sample size estimation for tests of hypotheses about classification probabilities, predictive probabilities, and diagnostic ratios will be introduced with a Bayesian focus. It is important to note that the sample size is constrained by practical limitations, including study cost and time constraints of the people involved. For example, in a busy university radiology department, scheduling of patients to undergo certain imaging techniques is always a problem because of the competing allocation of resources. The sample size will be based on the posterior probability of the alternative hypothesis, and previous knowledge of prior related studies is essential for successful study design. The investigator should be able to provide the statistician with a good guess of the future study results.

Only Bayesian principles will be used to estimate the sample size, thus, frequency concepts, such as power and Type I error, will not be invoked at this time.

5.7.2.1 Binary Tests

A Bayesian approach is taken for the selection of sample size. The usual ideas of Type I error and power will be avoided. Instead, the ideas of the posterior distribution of the parameters will be introduced. Therefore, the necessity for the Bayes theorem.

Suppose the population has a Bernoulli density, and let X be the number of successes in n trials, and suppose θ is the probability of a success on each trial, the density of X is then

$$f(x \mid \theta) \propto \theta^x (1 - \theta)^{n-x},$$

where $x = 0, 1, 2, \ldots, n$, and $0 \leq \theta \leq 1$.

If our information about θ is vague, we can use a uniform density for the parameter. This means the posterior density for θ is

$$f(x \mid \theta) \propto \theta^x (1 - \theta)^{n-x}, \quad 0 \leq \theta \leq 1.$$

This is considered as a function of θ and is a Beta distribution with parameters $a = x + 1$ and $b = n - x + 1$. All Bayesian inferences are based on this distribution. The mean of this distribution is

$$a/(a + b)$$

and the variance of θ is

$$(a/(a+b))(a/(a+b))(1/(a+b+1).$$

Note that $r = x/n$ is the proportion of successes in n trials.

We plan to select a random sample of size n from a Bernoulli population with θ as the population proportion. Let x be the number of successes and $r = x/n$ the sample proportion. The null hypothesis is

$$H\text{: } \theta \leq \theta_0 \text{ vs. } A\text{: } \theta \geq \theta_0$$

and the null hypothesis is rejected in favor of the alternative if

$$Pr(\theta \geq \theta_0 \mid n, x) = P, \tag{5.33}$$

where P is given. How is n selected so that Equation (5.33) is satisfied?

Obviously, we need information from the investigator, thus he or she is asked: In a future experiment, what do you expect the sample proportion r to be? Can you give a range of values for r? Alternatively, the experimenter could give us the results of previous related experiments reported as the number of successes in m past trials.

Note that Equation (5.33) can be verified if the posterior distribution of θ is known. As an example, consider

$$H\text{: } \theta < .2 \text{ vs. } A\text{: } \theta \geq .2,$$

where θ is the probability of the FPF of a binary diagnostic test. The historical rate of falsely declaring the test result as positive is 20%, and it is important to detect a FPF in excess of the historical rate. The clinical diagnostic radiologists believe the sample proportion r will vary from .22 to .30. What is the sample size? The null hypothesis is rejected if

$$Pr(\theta \geq .2 \mid r, n) = .9.$$

The sample proportion r is varied from .22 to .30, and n is varied over realistic values of the posterior probability P of the alternative hypothesis. The sample sizes vary in a reasonable way by increasing with rising values of P for a fixed r.

For example, if the future observed FPF is $r = .22$, $P = .939$, the required sample size is 1000, and the null hypothesis is rejected. On the other hand, when $r = .25$ and $P = .920$, the hypothesis is rejected with 100 patients. The sample size is decreasing with increasing r and only 25 patients are required when $r = .30$ in order to reject the null hypothesis.

See Table 5.14 for the sample sizes for various values of r and P. The values of r should represent what the experimenter reasonably expects to occur.

TABLE 5.14

Sample Sizes for FPF

r	a*	b*	a + b	P
r	*rn* + 1	(1 − *r*)*n* + 1	*n* + 2	?
.22	12	38	52	.712
.22	23	79	102	.704
.22	45	157	202	.779
.22	89	313	402	.886
.22	221	781	1002	.939
.25	13.5	38.5	52	.834
.25	26	74	102	.920
.25	51	151	202	.96
.25	126	376	502	.998
.30	4	8	12	.837
.30	8.5	18.5	27	.91
.30	31	71	102	.99
.35	10.45	18.55	29	.88

*a and b are the parameters of the Beta distribution.

When designing a Phase II developmental trial for a binary diagnostic test, both the FPF and TPF are taken into account in estimating the sample size. To do this, a joint credible region for the two-dimensional parameter (θ, ϕ) is used to test the null hypothesis H: $\theta \geq \theta_0$ or $\phi \leq \phi_0$ vs. the alternative A: $\theta < \theta_0$ and $\phi > \phi_0$ where θ is the probability of a false positive and ϕ the probability of a true positive. Therefore, the trial should answer the question: Is the false positive rate less than some specified amount θ_0, and does the true positive fraction exceed the value ϕ_0? For example, Pepe[6] examines the development of a diagnostic test for chlamydia where the test must have a sensitivity of at least .75 ($= \phi_0$) and a specificity of .80 ($1 - \theta_0$). How does the Bayesian address this problem? Table 5.15 presents several scenarios that depict various rates of false and true positives. For each row, the univariate and joint probabilities of the alternative hypothesis are computed. The joint probability is the posterior probability of the joint credible region, which is the Cartesian product of ($\theta < .2/data$) and ($\phi > .75/data$). Minitab was used

TABLE 5.15

Sample Sizes for a Binary Diagnostic Test

# Non diseased	# Diseased	# FP(%)	# TP(%)	P(θ < .2/*data*)	P(ϕ > .75/*data*)	Joint Probability
46	64	7(15.2)	51(79.6)	.584	.522	.334
46	64	5(10)	55(85)	.682	.752	.509
70	100	4(5.7)	91(91.2)	.870	.833	.719
46	64	1(2)	61(95)	.946	.934	.887*
100	150	2(2)	142(94.6)	.925	.929	.90
70	100	1(1.42)	95(95.6)	.976	.935	.912
150	200	3(2)	190(95)	.970	.952	.924

for this analysis, generating two columns, one for each parameter and each having a Beta distribution.

Suppose the null hypothesis is rejected when the joint probability is at least .85, then if 1 false positive occurs out of 46 nondiseased patients, and 61 true positive occur out of 64 diseased patients, the null hypothesis would be rejected with a probability of .887. The hypothetical FPF fraction is 2% and the hypothetical true positive fraction is 95%.

Comparing two binomial populations is a common problem in statistics and involves the null hypothesis H: $\theta_1 = \theta_2$ vs. the alternative A: $\phi_1 \neq \phi_2$ where θ_1 and θ_2 are parameters from two Bernoulli populations. The two Bernoulli parameters might be the sensitivities of two diagnostic modalities.

Assuming the prior probability of the null hypothesis is π and assigning independent uniform priors for the two Bernoulli parameters, it can be shown that the Bayesian test rejects H in favor of A if the posterior probability P of the alternative hypothesis satisfies

$$P > \gamma \tag{5.34}$$

where

$$P = D_2/D \tag{5.35}$$

and $D = D_1 + D_2$. It can be shown (see 4.26) that

$$D_1 = \left\{ \pi \binom{n_1}{x_1}\binom{n_2}{x_2} \Gamma(x_1 + x_2 + 1)\Gamma(n_1 + n_2 - x_1 - x_2 + 1) \right\} \div \Gamma(n_1 + n_2 + 2), \tag{5.36}$$

where Γ is the gamma function and

$$D_2 = (1 - \pi)(n_1 + 1)^{-1}(n_1 + 1)^{-1}.$$

X_1 and X_2 are the number of successes from the two binomial populations with parameters (θ_1, n_1) and (θ_2, n_2), respectively.

5.7.2.2 Multinomial Outcomes

Consider the mammography example with 60 patients given in Table 5.7. (See Section 5.3.5.)

In a previous section, it was shown that the ROC area is estimated as .768 (.091). Suppose the null hypothesis is H: auc = .7 vs. the alternative A: auc > .7, and that the null hypothesis is rejected if

$$P(\text{auc} > .7\ /\text{data}) > .90. \tag{5.37}$$

For the above outcomes, it can be shown that $P(\text{auc} > .7/\text{data}) = .778$, thus there is not sufficient evidence to reject the null hypothesis. Suppose the

TABLE 5.16

Alternative Mammogram Test Results I

Status	Normal (1)	Benign (2)	Probably Benign (3)	Suspicious (4)	Malignant (5)	Total
Cancer	0	0	5	13	12	30
No Cancer	11	8	7	4	0	30

outcomes would have been as shown in Table 5.16. Do these outcomes provide enough evidence to reject the null hypothesis? It can be shown the ROC area is .852(.066) and that $P(\text{auc} > .7/\text{data}) = .976$, therefore the null would be rejected. As the estimated ROC area increases, the probability of the alternative hypothesis increases for the same sample size. On the other hand, suppose the outcomes would have been as seen in Table 5.17? Then, the estimated ROC area is .371(.174) and $P(\text{auc} > .7/\text{data}) = .050$, consequently, the null hypothesis would not be rejected. The above shows the effect of the estimated ROC area on the probability of rejecting the null hypothesis. Note the sample size was the same for all scenarios.

5.7.3 Sample Sizes: Continuous Diagnostic Scores

When the diagnostic score is continuous, there are several approaches to estimating the ROC area, such as: (1) the binormal model, (2) the nonparametric approach, and (3) using an exponential distribution for the scores. The binormal approach will be used here, but the reader is referred to Zhou et al.[2] and to Pepe[6] for descriptions of nonparametric procedures, including the Mann–Whitney U-Test. Hanley and McNeil[15] estimate the ROC based on an exponential distribution for the diagnostic scores, and Hanley[16] provides a good introduction.

In what is to follow, sample size estimates are introduced for estimating and testing hypotheses about one ROC area; this is followed by a Bayesian approach to finding the sample sizes in order to compare two ROC areas.

5.7.3.1 One ROC Curve

The binormal model for the ROC curve is based on a normal distribution for the diagnostic scores of the independent diseased and nondiseased populations.

TABLE 5.17

Alternative Mammogram Test Results II

Status	Normal (1)	Benign (2)	Probably Benign (3)	Suspicious (4)	Malignant (5)	Total
Cancer	9	2	11	8	0	30
No Cancer	1	0	6	11	12	30

Let us consider a random sample $x_i = (x_{i1}, x_{i2}, \ldots, x_{in_i})$ of size n_i ($i = 1, 2$) from a normal $(\mu_i, 1/\tau_i)$ population where $\tau_i = 1/\sigma_i^2$ is the inverse of the variance, and suppose the prior information is vague and that Jeffrey's prior $\xi(\mu_i, \tau_i) \propto 1/\tau_i$ is appropriate, then the posterior density of the parameters is

$$\xi(\mu_i, \tau_i \,/\, data) \propto \tau_i^{n_i/2-1} \exp-(\tau_i/2)\left[n_i(\mu_i - \bar{x}_i)^2 + (n_i - 1)S_i^2\right]. \tag{5.38}$$

From this, it follows that the posterior distribution of μ_i/τ_i is normal with mean $\bar{x}_i$ and precision $n_i\tau_i$ and that the marginal posterior distribution of τ_i is gamma with parameters $a_i = (n_i - 1)/2$ and $b_i = (n_i - 1)S_i^2/2$ where S_i^2 is the sample variance.

It can be shown that the area under the ROC curve is given by

$$A(\mu_1, \mu_2, \tau_1, \tau_2 / data) = \Phi\ [(\mu_2 - \mu_1)/(1/\tau_1 + 1/\tau_2)], \tag{5.39}$$

where Φ is the CDF of the standard normal distribution. The subscript 2 labels the diseased population, and the subscript 1 denotes the nondiseased population. To summarize, assuming a vague prior density for the parameters, the posterior distribution of the population mean and precision is normal gamma. Therefore, the posterior distribution of the ROC area is induced by the posterior distribution of the four population parameters. The Bayesian approach to estimating the ROC area is based on the so-called binormal assumption. Note that the ROC area AUC depends on the unknown parameters of the model. Bayesian methods for estimating the ROC area will be illustrated by referring to an example found in Zhou et al. that is based on the study by Hans et al.[12] The data are given in Table 4.12 of Zhou et al. and refer to the use of CK-BB, an enzyme in the spinal fluid collected within 24 hours of injury to predict the outcome of severe trauma. (This example was also used in Section 5.4.)

There are 60 patients and 19 do not have severe trauma. The 41 patients who had a poor outcome have a mean CK-BB level of 427.29 with a standard deviation of 372.63, while for those 19 patients with a good outcome, the mean CK-BB level was 151.5 with a standard deviation of 91.11.

Below are the program statements for the Bayesian estimation of the area under the ROC curve based on the posterior distribution of the four population parameters.

```
model
# Zhou et al head trauma
{ area <- phi((mu2-mu1)/sqrt(1/tau1 + 1/tau2))
# based on formula (5.39)
# mu2 is mean of patients with poor outcome
# vague prior density for the mean and precision
mu1~ dnorm(117.52, prec1)
# mu1 is mean of patients with a good outcome
```

```
mu2~dnorm (427.29, prec2)
prec1<-n1*tau1
prec2<-n2*tau2
# tau1 is precision of those with good outcome
tau1~dgamma( a1,b1)
# tau2 is precision of those with poor outcome
tau2 ~dgamma(a2,b2)
# binormal parameters
a<-(mu2-mu1)*sqrt(tau2)
b<-sqrt(tau2/tau1)
c<-step(area-.80)
}
list( n1= 19, n2=41, a1=9, b1= 74709.28, a2= 20, b2=
2777062.33)
list( mu1= 0, mu2= 0,  tau1 =1, tau2 =1)
```

To show the effect of sample size on inference, two basic scenarios are used: (1) the sample sizes are increased by a factor of 4, keeping the sample means and standard deviations constant at the levels found in the original study to determine the effect of estimating the area (Table 5.18A), and (2) increasing the mean level of CK-BB for those with a poor outcome from 427 to 527 and increasing the sample size by a factor of 4 to see the effect on the probability of the alternative hypothesis, $P(\text{area} > .80/\text{data})$ (Table 5.18B).

These results show that when the sample size is increased by a factor of 4, the standard deviation of the posterior distribution of the area decreases by a factor of 2. Of course, the same result would be obtained with the frequency properties of the sample mean.

In this case, the sample mean of those with poor outcome was increased from 427 to 527, resulting in a posterior mean area of about .85. Suppose the null hypothesis is that H: auc < .8 vs. the alternative that A: auc > .8, and H is rejected if

$$P(\text{auc} > .8/\text{data}) > .90,$$

TABLE 5.18A

Sample Size for Estimating the ROC Area

n_1	n_2	Area	SD	Interval
5	10	.763	.108	.52, .93
19	41	.784	.052	.67, .87
76	164	.787	.026	.73, .84
304	656	.789	.013	.76, .81

TABLE 5.18B

Sample Sizes for Testing Hypothesis

n_1	n_2	Area	SD	Interval	P(area > .8/data)
5	10	.842	.091	.62, .97	.720
19	41	.850	.045	.74, .92	.862
76	164	.856	.022	.80, .89	.989
304	656	.857	.011	.83, .87	1.00

then, 76 patients with a good outcome (with a sample mean CK-BB level of 117.52 and standard deviation of 91.11) and 164 patients with a poor outcome (mean level 527, with a standard deviation of 327) would be sufficient to reject the null hypothesis. It is important to note that the sample means and standard deviations of the patients in the two groups should be chosen with care and based on previous related studies. Thus, the choice of 527 as the sample mean of CK-BB for those with a poor outcome should be reasonably expected to occur in a future study.

5.7.3.2 *Two ROC Curves*

The following program statements compute the ROC areas under the curve for two independent diagnostic tests comparing the diagnostic accuracy for the head trauma information considered above and taken from Zhou et al.[2] This is an obvious expansion of the previous WinBUGS program and is somewhat hypothetical in that, for the second group, the mean CK-BB level for the patients with a good outcome is the same (117.52, with a standard deviation of 91.11) as that in the original study; however, the mean level for those with a poor outcome increased from 427.29 (with a standard deviation of 372.63) to 527.29 (with a standard deviation of 372.63). The sample sizes for the two groups are the same as in the original study, namely 41 with a good outcome and 19 with a poor one.

With this sample size, what is the difference in the two areas? To answer this question, suppose the null hypothesis is

$$H\text{: } a < .025 \text{ vs. the alternative } A\text{: } a > .025$$

where *a is* the absolute value of the difference in the two ROC areas. See the relevant statement below, namely *a* < –*abs*(*diff*). The posterior probability of the alternative hypothesis is

$$P(a > .025/\text{data}) = .826.$$

The statement *b* < –step(*a*– .025) calculates this probability and the MCMC procedure is based on 25,000 simulations with a refreshing rate of 500. Is this sufficient evidence to reject the null hypothesis? On the other hand,

$$P(\ a > .05/\text{data}) = .648$$

and

$$P(a > .10/\text{data}) = .333,$$

which puts the statement $P(a > .025/\text{data}) = .826$ into perspective. It can also be shown that the estimated areas of the two groups are .784 (.053) and .853 (.044), respectively.

```
Model;
{
auc1 <- phi((mu2-mu1)/sqrt(1/p1 + 1/p2))
auc2 <- phi((vu2-vu1)/sqrt(1/q1 + 1/q2))
diff <-auc1-auc2
mu1~dnorm(117.52,prec1)
mu2~dnorm(427.29,prec2)
# mu1 is mean CB-KK level for those with good outcome
of group 1
# mu2 is mean CB-KK level for those with a poor outcome
of group 1
# prec1 is the precision of those with good outcome
group 1
# prec2 is precision of those with a poor outcome group1
prec1<-n1*p1
prec2<-n2*p2
vu1~ dnorm( 117.52 ,qrec1)
vu2 ~dnorm(527.29 ,qrec2)
# vu 1 is mean level with a good outcome of group 2
# vu 2 is mean level with a poor outcome of group 2
# qrec1 is the precision of those with good outcome
group 2
# qrec2 is precision of those with a poor outcome group
2
qrec1<-m1*q1
qrec2<-m2
p1~dgamma(a1,b1)
p2~dgamma(a2,b2)
q1~dgamma(e1,f1)
q2~dgamma(e2,f2)
a<-abs(diff)
b<-step(a-.025)
```

```
c<-step(a-.05)
d<-step(a-.10)

}

list(n1=19, n2= 41, a1 = 9, b1= 74709.28, a2= 20, b2 =
2777062.33,m1=19 ,m2 = 41, e1= 9.5, f1= 74709.28, e2=
20.5, f2 = 2777062.33)
list( mu1= 0, mu2= 0,vu1= 0,vu2= 0,
p1=1,p2=1,q1=1,q2=1)
```

5.8 Exercises

5.1. Verify Equation (5.12).

5.2. Using Equation (5.12), find the ROC area for the Spokane Heart Study. (See Section 5.4.2.)

5.3. How would one estimate the proportion of ties $P(Y = Z)$ in the scores of the normal and abnormal ROIs for the clustered mammography data. Use Equation (5.23).

5.4. Refer to Section 5.6. Does the Bayesian analysis agree with the conventional analysis of Pepe[6]?

   a. The two ROC areas are based on 4 (including (0,0) and (1,1)) points of the ROC curve. Is the first underestimating the area? Is the second overestimating the area? Why?

   b. What is the analysis for unpaired data? Assume two independent groups. What is the estimate of $P(Y = Z)$? Test the H: rsp(CPH,ETS) > 1 vs. A: rsp(CPH,ETS) < 1.

   c. Verify Table 5.13.

5.5. See Section 5.7.2.1 and Table 5.14. Develop a scenario with a FPF = 10% and a TPF = 85%, and find the sample size that gives a joint posterior probability of .80. How does your result compare to Pepe?

5.6. See Equation (5.36) of Section 5.7.2.1. Find the sample size (the number of diseased patients) for testing the null hypothesis H: $\theta_1 = \theta_2$ vs. the alternative A: $\theta_1 \neq \theta_2$ where θ_1 and the θ_2 are the sensitivities of two diagnostic tests. Assume equal number ($n_1 = n_2$) of subjects in two groups and reject H whenever

$$P(\theta_1 \neq \theta_2 / n_1, n_2, x_1, x_2) = .90.$$

TABLE 5.19

Mammography Test Results for Problem 5.7

Status	Normal (1)	Benign (2)	Probably Benign (3)	Suspicious (4)	Malignant (5)	Total
Cancer	0	0	0	12	18	30
No Cancer	18	8	4	0	0	30

Assume the two groups of patients are independent. Find the sample sizes assuming the two sample sensitivities (the fraction of patients with a positive test results) are .70 and .90, respectively, for groups 1 and 2. Also assume, *a priori*, that the probability of the null hypothesis is .5 and that, under the alternative hypothesis, the prior densities of the sensitivities are uniform over (0,1).

5.7. See Section 5.7.2.2. Suppose the outcomes for mammography are what is shown in Table 5.19:

   a. What is the estimated ROC area using the Bayesian approach?
   b. Using the criterion

$$P(\text{ auc} > .7 \;/\; \text{data}) > .98,$$

   will the null hypothesis be rejected?

   c. As the test scores increase, does the probability of breast cancer decrease? Explain.

5.8. Verify Equation (5.39).

5.9. Verify Table 5.18A and Table 5.18B. What is the estimation error in estimating the mean ROC area for 82 patients with a poor outcome and 38 with a good outcome? Assume the sample means and variances are the same as those used in Table 5.18A.

5.10. See Table 5.18A Fewer patients (< 76 with a good outcome and < 164 with a poor outcome) could be used to reject the null hypothesis. Find a smaller number of patients in each that would be sufficient. What is the smallest number in each group? Use the program associated with the table.

5.11. See Section 5.7.3.2. The above scenario assumes the two groups are independent; however, in practice, it is more likely that the two groups are dependent, as in the case of two readers. Write a WinBUGS program to cover this situation and explore the effect of sample size on the posterior probability of absolute difference in the two correlated ROC areas.

5.12. Derive the formula: AUC $= \Phi[a/\sqrt{1+b^2}\,]$, where X is normally distributed, $a = (\mu_D - \mu_{\bar{D}})/\sigma_D$, and $b = \sigma_D/\sigma_{\bar{D}}$. The mean and standard deviation of the X for the diseased population are μ_D and σ_D, respectively, while $\mu_{\bar{D}}$ and $\sigma_{\bar{D}}$ are the mean and standard deviation of X for the nondiseased. Φ is the cumulative distribution function of the standard normal distribution.

References

1. Obuchowski, N.A., Lieber, M.L, and Powell, K.A., Data analysis for detection and localization of multiple abnormalities with application to mammography, *Acad. Radiol.*, 7:516, 2000.
2. Zhou, H.H., McClish, D.K., and Obuchowski, N.A., *Statistical Methods for Diagnostic Medicine*, John Wiley & Sons, 2002, New York.
3. Bogaert, J., Kuzo, R., Dymarkowski, S., Becker, R., Piessens, J., and Rademakers, F.E., Coronary artery imaging with real-time navigator three-dimensional turbo field echo MR coronary angiography: initial experience, *Radiology*, 226, 707, 2003.
4. Theate, F.L., Fuhrman, C.R., Oliver, J.H., et al., Digital radiography and conventional imaging of the chest: a comparison of observer performance, *Am. J. Roentgeneol.*, 162, 575,1994.
5. Beam, C.A., Lyde, P.M., and Sullivan, D.C., Variability in the interpretation of screening mammograms by U.S. radiologists, *Arch. Int. Med.*, 156, 209, 1996.
6. Pepe, M.S., *The Statistical Evaluation of Medical Tests for Classification and Prediction*, Oxford University Press, 2003, Oxford, U.K.
7. Broemeling, L.D., *The Bayesian Analysis of Linear Models*, Marcel Dekker, 1985, New York.
8. Wiener, D.A., Ryan, T.J., McCabe, C.H., Kennedy, J.W., Schloss, M., Tristani, F., Chaitman, B.R., and Fisher, L.D., Correlations among history of angina, ST-segmented response and prevalence of coronary artery disease, *N. Engl. J. Med.*, 301, 230, 1979.
9. Mielke, H.C., Shields, P.J., and Broemeling, L.D., Coronary artery calcium scores for men and women of a large asymptomatic population, *Cardiovas. Dis. Preven.*, 2, 194, 1999.
10. Rumberger, J.A., Brundage, B.H., Rader, D.J., and Kondos, G., Electron beam computed tomographic coronary calcium scanning: a review and guidelines for use in asymptomatic patients, *Mayo Clin. Proc.*, 74, 243, 1999.
11. Egan, J.P., *Signal Detection Theory and ROC Analysis*, Academic Press, 1975, New York.
12. Hans, P., Albert, A., Born, D., and Chapelle, J.P., Derivation of a biochemical prognostic index in severe head injury, *Intens. Care Med.*, 11, 186, 1985.
13. O'Malley, J.A., Zou, K.H., Fielding, J.R., and Tampany, C.M.C., Bayesian regression methodology for estimating a receiver operating characteristic curve with two radiologic applications: prostate biopsy and spiral CT of ureteral stones, *Acad. Radiol.*, 8, 713, 2001.
14. Somoza, E. and Mossman, D. "Biological Markers" and psychiatric diagnosis: risk-benefit balancing using ROC analysis, *Biol. Psych.*, 29, 811,1991.
15. Hanley, J.A. and McNeil, B.J., The meaning and use of the area under a receiver operating characteristic curve, *Radiology*, 143, 29, 1982.
16. Hanley, J.A., Receiver operating characteristic (ROC) methodology: the state of the art, *Crit. Rev. Diagn. Imag.* , 29, 307,1989.

Chapter 6

Regression and Test Accuracy

6.1 Introduction

It is well known that test accuracy depends on many factors, including differences in readers and differences in various patient characteristics. For example, the age of the patient, their gender, the stage of the disease, and the therapy received, all have a bearing on the measured test accuracy. This chapter describes Bayesian regression procedures for estimating the effect of patient and reader covariates on test accuracy, as measured by classification probabilities, predictive probabilities, and diagnostic likelihood ratios. In the case of quantitative diagnostic scores, regression techniques will be used to allow for these patient and reader characteristics when estimating the ROC area. For additional information on this, refer to Pepe[1] (Chaps. 3 and 6) and to Zhou et al.[2] (Chap. 8).

In the following, Bayesian regression techniques for binary test scores will be illustrated with an audiology example taken from Leisenring et al.[3] and also analyzed by Pepe. In this example, the probability of a false positive on the hearing test of the ear of a patient is regressed on patient covariates, including age, severity of disease, and location of the hearing test. Two modeling approaches are taken: (1) using the log linear function illustrated by Pepe, and (2) using a logistic link function. By way of contrast and comparison, a nonBayesian analysis is also presented for the audiology study. In addition, the effect of patient covariates on other measures of test accuracy, including true positive fraction and the positive diagnostic likelihood ratio, are examined with regression techniques using log and logit link functions.

Two additional examples estimate the effect of patients' covariates on a continuous test result. The first example determines the effect of gender on response to therapy for lung cancer, then uses that information to examine the effect on the area under the receiving operating characteristic (ROC) curve. The second example involves the measurement of prostate specific antigen to diagnose prostate cancer and investigates the effect of age on properties of the ROC curve.

6.2 Audiology Study

6.2.1 Introduction

The dataset for this study can be downloaded at *http://www.fhcrc.org/labs/pepe/book* and is analyzed extensively in Pepe. Earlier various analyses appear in Leisenring et al.[3–5] It comprises 3152 cases where the experimental unit is an ear. There were three modalities (diagnostic tests a, b, and c) and each hearing test took place in either a room or booth. The result was binary with 1690 tests being designated as positive (hearing impaired) and 1460 being designated as not hearing impaired. According to the gold standard, 1256 ears were indeed impaired, while 1896 were not impaired. Other patient covariates were age and disease severity.

Among the tests, 1039 were given test a, 1053 were given test b, and 1060 test c. Among the 1039 ears receiving test a, 515 were administered in a room and 524 in a booth. Also, 633 were declared normal according to the gold standard, while the remaining 406 were designated hearing impaired. Among the 633 who were declared to have normal ears, the number of false positives that occurred was 253, with 380 true negative.

6.2.2 Log Link Function

The analysis for this data appears in Pepe[1](p. 54) where the true positive occurrence is modeled with a generalized linear model using a log link function with age, location (room or booth), and severity of disease as patient covariates. There are 253 false positives among the 633 normal ears given test a.

The log link model is

$$\phi = \exp(\alpha_1 + \alpha_2 x_1 + \alpha_3 x_2)$$

where ϕ is the probability of a false positive, x_1 is the age of the patient, and x_2 indicates the location where $x_2 = 1$ for a booth and $x_2 = 0$ for a room. The program statements follow.

```
model
{
( for( i in 1 : N ) {
r[i] ~ dbern(p[i])
p[i]<- exp(alpha[1] + alpha[2] * x1 [i]+alpha
[3]*x2[i])
}

phat <- mean(p[])
for (i in 1:3){
```

```
beta[i] ~ dnorm(0.0,0.0001)}
e <-exp(alpha[2])
f <-exp(alpha[3])
}
```

TABLE 6.1

Posterior Distribution of Audiology Study

Parameter	Mean	SD	2.5%	Median	97.5%
e	1.008	.0089	.9888	1.008	1.028
f	1.194	.119	.98	1.188	1.445
alpha[1]	−1.303	.368	−2.037	−1.296	−0.5869
alpha[2]	.0081	.0097	−.0112	.00807	.0274
alpha[3]	.1725	.0994	−.0202	.1719	.3683
phat	.1973	.0095	.1787	.1972	.2163

The *r* vector is the occurrence of false positives (1 indicates a false positive and 0 indicates a true negative). The vector x_1 contains the age of a patient and the vector of locations (room or booth) is x_2. The vector of false positive probabilities is given by p[], and the alpha coefficients are the regression parameters on the log scale. These parameters are given a vague normal prior with mean 0.0 and precision 0.0001. The main parameter is f, which estimates the ratio of the false positive rate of a booth to that of a room. The number of samples generated was 25,000, and 100 observations were refreshed. The Bayesian analysis is given in Table 6.1.

Age has little effect on the probability of a false positive; however, as for location, the ratio of the false positive fraction of a booth to the false positive fraction of a room is estimated as 1.194 with a 95% credible interval of (.98, 1.445). This estimate is adjusted for age. How does this compare to Pepe's analysis (Table 3.9, on p. 54)? The estimate of f is 1.18, with a 95% confidence interval of (.96, 1.46), which is quite close to the Bayesian, which is not a surprising result because the Bayesian analysis employed a vague prior for the model parameters. The observed estimate of the false positive rate for a booth is 134/310 = 0.432 compared to 119/323 = 0.368 for a room, thus the raw ratio of booth to room is 1.1739. In order to compare the other parameters between the Bayesian and the Pepe analysis, see Table 6.1 and Pepe (Table 3.9.) Note that phat is the estimate of the overall false positive rate for the normal ears and is estimated as 0.1973. To run this program, the data must be imported from the worksheet provided in the downloaded file, which can be accessed from the Internet address given above.

6.2.3 Logistic Link

Another plausible approach to assessing the effect of patient covariates on the false positive rate is with the logistic link function that appears in the WinBUGS® program below:

```
model
{
for(i in1:N) {
r[i] ~ dbern(p[i])
logit(p[i])<- beta[1] + beta[2] *
x4[i]+beta[3]*x2[i]+beta[4]*x2[i]*x4[i]
}
phat <- mean(p[])
for (i in 1:4)
beta[i] ~ dnorm(0.0,0.0001)}
e<-exp(beta[2])
f<-exp(beta[3])
g<-exp(beta[4])
}
```

The r vector is as before, the vector of false positive occurrences among ears given the hearing test a or b, x_2 is the vector of locations (room or booth), and x_4 (= 1 for test a and 0 for test b) is the indicator vector for test mode. The logistic link is quite natural as a model for binary information such as the occurrence of a false positive, and has the advantage over the log link in that, with the latter, the false positive rate might exceed the value 1. On the other hand, the interpretation of the model parameters is somewhat more complex with the logistic link, that is, with the logistic, one employs odds ratios, while with the log link, interpretation of the model coefficient is as a ratio of probabilities.

We now return to a different aspect of the audiology example, which was described by Pepe[1] (Table 3.12, p. 57). Here, the false positive occurrence was regressed on the test modality (a vs. b), the location (room vs. booth), and the location by test interaction. The later interaction estimates the odds ratio of a false positive for test a vs. b for a booth compared to the odds ratio of a false positive of test a vs. test b for a room. This interaction effect is estimated by the exp(beta[4]) = g in the above listing of program statements. In this program, one must import the three vectors r, x_2, and x_4 into the worksheet above from the Internet address. The regression coefficients are given vague prior normal distributions and phat estimates the overall false positive rate among those ears receiving tests a and b hearing modalities. The logistic Bayesian analysis provided the posterior results depicted in Table 6.2.

Regarding *g* as the main parameter of interest, the odds ratio of a booth vs. the odds ratio for a room is estimated as 1.434, and the corresponding credible interval is (.8817, 2.21) and, of course, this is an adjusted estimate. Therefore, the odds ratio for a booth is 43% larger compared to the odds ratio for a room. The graph of the posterior density of *g* is shown in Figure 6.1. The simulation used 24,500 observations from the posterior distribution of *g*, while refreshing with 500 observations.

TABLE 6.2

Posterior Distribution of False Positive Rate

Parameter	Mean	SD	2.5%	Median	97.5%
e	.9878	.1627	.7115	.9746	1.346
f	.9457	.167	.6735	.9331	1.29
g	1.434	.339	.8817	1.395	2.21
beta[1]	−.513	.1142	−.7411	−.513	−.2902
beta[2]	−.0255	.1633	−.3404	−.0257	.2971
beta[3]	−.0695	.1652	−.3953	−.0692	.2543
beta[4]	.3333	.2337	−.1295	.3328	.793
phat	.3833	.0135	.3568	.3831	.4106

6.2.4 Diagnostic Likelihood Ratio

The positive diagnostic likelihood ratio was briefly discussed in Section 5.3.4 and is defined as

$$\text{PDLR} = \text{TPF}/\text{FPF} \tag{6.1}$$

where TPF is the true positive fraction and FPF is the false positive fraction. Thus, if

$$\log(\text{TPF}) = \text{beta}[1] + \text{beta}[2]X$$

and

$$\log(\text{FPF}) = \text{alpha}[1] + \text{alpha}[2]X$$

where X is the indictor function for test a or b ($X = 1$ for test a and 0 for test b), then

$$\log(\text{PDLR}) = \text{beta}[1] - \text{alpha}[1] + (\text{beta}[2] - \text{alpha}[2])X \tag{6.2}$$

and exp(beta[2] – alpha[2]) is the ratio of the positive diagnostic likelihood ratios (PDLRs) for test a relative to test b. The TPF is estimated from the diseased patients and the FPF from only the nondiseased.

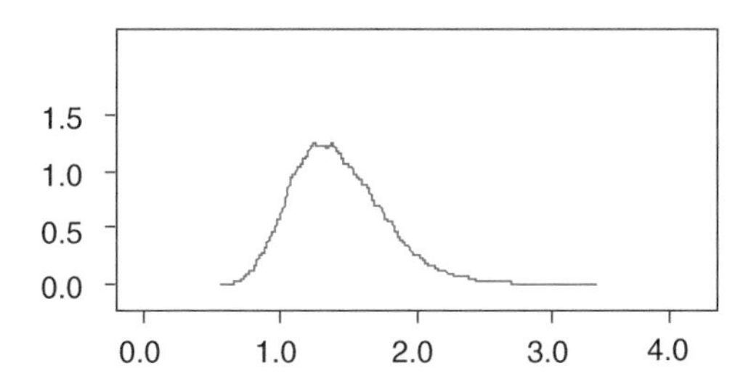

FIGURE 6.1
Posterior Distribution of *g*.

TABLE 6.3

Posterior Distribution of the Positive Diagnostic Likelihood Ratio Audiology Example

Parameter	Mean	SD	2.5%	Median	97.5%
alpha[1]	−1.547	.1273	−1.786	−1.557	−1.282
alpha[2]	1.382	.1296	1.105	1.392	1.621
beta[1]	−1.005	.052	−1.111	−1.004	−.9053
beta[2]	.08506	.07002	−.04601	.0839	.2214
fphat	.3826	.01357	.3565	.3828	.4088
tphat	.6016	.01625	.5727	.6043	.6369
pdlr	1.582	.07094	1.45	1.58	1.725
rpdlrab	3.696	.5355	2.641	3.688	4.795

Below is the program for estimating the PDLR and the effect of the test modality (test a or b) on the PDLR. The program below can be typed directly onto the WinBUGS worksheet and executed. There are 529 hearing impaired ears with information on the true positive status (given by the tp ((true positive)) vector), along with the matched information on test a or b (given by the x_4 vector). With regard to the false positive information, there are 1276 normal ears with false positive information indicated by the vector fp (false positive) and the corresponding information on the occurrence of test a or test b, given by the vector x_5. There are two parameters of interest, namely PDLR and the ratio of the PDLR for test a relative to test b. The results of running the program are given in Table 6.3.

```
model
{
for( i in 1 : M ) {
fp[i] ~ dbern(p[i])
p[i] <- exp(beta[1] + beta[2] * x5[i])
}
for(i in 1:N) { tp[i]~dbern(q[i])
q[i]<-exp(alpha[1]+alpha[2]*x4[i])
}
tphat<-mean(q[])
fphat <- mean(p[])
for (i in 1:2 ){

beta[i] ~ dnorm(0.0,0.0001)
alpha[i] ~dnorm(0.0,0.0001)
}
a<-exp(alpha[2])
```

```
b<-exp(beta[2])
rpdlrab <- exp(alpha[2]-beta[2])
pdlr<-tphat/fphat
}
```

What does this tell us about the effect of test modality on the value of the positive diagnostic likelihood ratio? The average value over test a and test b is 1.58, with a 95% credible interval of 1.45 to 1.725. On the other hand, the ratio of the PDLR for test a relative to test b is given by RPDLRAB and has a posterior mean of 3.696, that is, the average value of the positive diagnostic ratio for test a is 3.69 times the PDLR for test b.

6.3 ROC Area and Patient Covariates

6.3.1 Introduction

When the diagnostic scores are binary, the accuracy is measured by sensitivity and specificity; however, when they are continuous, the acknowledged method of determining accuracy is with the area under the ROC curve. If the diagnostic score is continuous, the score could be dichotomized, and the sensitivity and specificity estimated; however, this could result in a loss of information leading to estimates of test accuracy that are unreliable. When the continuous score is dichotomized, the threshold value must be chosen with care, as we have seen in previous chapters.

As with binary scores, patient covariate effects on the diagnostic score should be taken into account when estimating the area under the ROC curve. The problem of assessing the effect of covariates on the ROC curve was first considered by Tosteson and Begg[6] for ordinal data, but was later generalized to continuous scores by Toledano and Gatsonis.[7] For a good introduction to the subject, see Pepe[1] (Chap. 6), who presents several methods of incorporating patient covariate information into the ROC curve. She describes nonparametric, semiparametric, and parametric regression methods to estimate the ROC area.

For the binormal model (assuming the diagnostic scores are normally distributed), the induced ROC curve technique of regressing the diagnostic score on covariates will be adopted for the Bayesian approach taken here.

Two examples are used to illustrate the effect of patient covariates on the ROC curve. First, an example taken from Holtbrugge and Schumacher[8] demonstrates the effect of gender on the ROC area. It is a clinical study of two therapies for lung cancer and was analyzed from a Bayesian viewpoint by Gregurich,[9] who developed an ordinal regression technique based on a generalized least squares concept to compare the two therapies. The diagnostic score is the response to therapy, measured on a four-point ordinal scale. The area under the ROC curve measures the separation between the two therapy patient groups. The second example is taken from a study of

Etzioni et al.[10] about the effect of age on prostate specific antigen (PSA) and, consequently, on the area of the ROC curve. The latter investigation is further examined in Pepe. A simple WinBUGS program performs a regression of the diagnostic score on patient covariates and disease status to see how the ROC area is affected. The same program also estimates the area under the curve.

6.3.2 ROC Curve as Response to Therapy

The Holtbrugge and Schumacher[8] study was a clinical trial with two therapeutic strategies where the treatments were compared with respect to tumor response. The sequential therapy method was used in the first group, who were given the same combination of agents, while the second group was given an alternating approach with three different combinations of agents alternating from cycle to cycle. The tumor response was assessed at the end of treatment as: progressive disease, no change, partial remission, and complete remission. The Table 6.4 provides the outcomes.

TABLE 6.4

Tumor Response

Therapy	Gender	Progressive Disease	No Change	Partial Remission	Complete Remission	Total
Sequential	Male	28	45	29	26	128
	Female	4	12	5	2	23
Total		32	57	34	28	151
Alternating	Male	41	44	20	20	125
	Female	12	7	3	1	23
Total		53	51	23	21	148

Gregurich[9] analyzed the results with a Bayesian regression model for ordinal data utilizing a generalized least squares approach. Our approach will be to estimate the ROC area using the induced method where the tumor response is regressed on gender and disease status with the program below. The effect of gender on tumor response is assessed first and, if the effect is "significant," gender specific ROC areas can be estimated. From Table 6.4, two columns, d and sex, can be constructed for input to the program.

```
model;
# Calculates the induced ROC curve
# Holtbrugge and Schumacher (1991) trial
{
# likelihood function
for(i in 1:N) {
y[i]~ dnorm(mu[i],precy[d[i]+1]);
mu[i] <- beta[1] + beta[2]*d[i] + beta[3]*sex[i] +
beta[4]*sex[i]*d[i];
```

```
}# prior distributions - noninformative prior;
similarly for informative priors
for(i in 1:P) {
beta[i] ~ dnorm(0, 0.000001);
}
for(i in 1:K) {
precy[i]~dgamma(0.001, 0.001);
vary[i] <- 1.0/precy[i];}
# calculates area under the curve
a <- beta[2]/sqrt(vary[2]); # ROC curve parameters
la2 <- vary[1]/vary[2];
auc <- phi(a/sqrt(1+la2))
b<- sqrt(la2)
```

The regression of Y on gender, disease, and the interaction between gender and disease is

$$Y = \text{beta}[1] + \text{beta}[2]*\text{d} + \text{beta}[3]*\text{sex} + \text{beta}[4]*\text{d}*\text{sex} + \sigma_d * \varepsilon \qquad (6.3)$$

where $\sigma_d = \sigma_1 I(d = 1) + \sigma_0 I(d = 0)$, and $\varepsilon \sim N(0,1)$. When d = 0 sequential therapy is indicated, and d = 1 the alternating, while sex = 0 indicates female, and sex = 1, male. Note that Y (= 1,2,3,4) is the response variable where 1, 2, 3, 4 indicate progressive disease, no change, partial remission, and complete response, respectively.

The induced ROC curve is

$$ROC_{sex} = \Phi[beta[2]/\sigma_1 + beta[4]/\sigma_1 * sex + (\sigma_0/\sigma_1)\Phi^{-1}(1 - t)] \qquad (6.4)$$

where Φ is the standard normal CDF (cumulative distribution function) and t is the false positive fraction. This curve is covariate specific and depends on the value of the covariate sex = 0 or 1, but if beta[4] is zero, the covariate has no effect on the ROC curve. Therefore, the approach is to first assess the importance of the covariate, and if it is significant, estimate the ROC area for different levels of the covariate. The estimated induced curve parameters are given in Table 6.5.

The 95% credible interval for beta[4] is (–.3884, .909), which is evidence that the covariate sex has a minimal effect on the ROC curve. Covariate specific ROC curve areas were estimated with a posterior mean of .546 (.035) for males and .552 (.080) for females, demonstrating that gender has little effect on separating the effect of therapy. The posterior variances for the two groups are not very different.

TABLE 6.5

Posterior Distribution of Induced ROC curve

Parameter	Mean	SD	2.5%	Median	9.75%
beta[1]	3.305	.2158	2.882	3.304	3.73
beta[2	−.5325	.305	−1.123	−.5328	.0669
beta[3	−.4571	.2347	−.92	−.4557	−.001503
beta[4]	.2605	.3314	−.3884	.261	.909
Vary0	1.077	.1281	.8538	1.067	1.354
Vary1	1.054	.1237	.8381	1.045	1.321

6.3.3 Diagnosing Prostate Cancer

In Etzione et al.,[10] 683 patients had their prostate specific antigen levels measured for screening of prostate cancer and it was found that 454 did not have the disease and 229 did. To download this dataset: *http://www.fhcrc.org/labs/pepe/book* and see Pepe[1] for the details of this study. Patient covariates included age where the average age among those without the disease was 64.8 and those with disease was also 64.8 years. Among those with prostate cancer, the total prostate specific antigen (PSA) was 10.31 mg/dL, and was 2.02 mg/dL among those without. The total PSA measurements were highly skewed to the right with mean and median levels of 2.02 and 1.31, respectively, for those without disease, but were 10.31 and 4.39, respectively, for those with cancer. It was decided to take logarithms of the total PSA levels for a binomial analysis. Also, for many subjects, repeated measurements of total PSA levels were taken, but this was not considered a covariate. The regression of log total PSA levels on disease status (d = 0,1), age, and the age by disease interaction gave the posterior analysis shown in Table 6.6.

The 95% credible interval for the age by disease interaction is (−.0372, .0126), which suggests that age has a minimal effect on the ROC curve. Adjusting for age, the ROC area was estimated at .9053 with a 95% credible interval of (.625, .997).

TABLE 6.6

Regression of PSA on Disease Status and Age

Parameter	Effect	Mean	SD	2.5%	Median	97.5%
beta[1]		−2.399	.1066	.6253	.9391	−1.559
beta[2]	Disease	2.056	.829	.4263	2.056	3.681
beta[3]	Age	.4256	.0062	.03025	.04261	.0548
beta[4]	Age by disease interaction	−.0123	.0127	−.0372	−.0123	.0126
vary0	Variance of nondiseased	.5375	.0359	.4716	.5359	.6129
vary1	Variance of diseased	1.232	.116	1.023	1.225	1.48
auc	area	.9053	.1006	.6253	.9391	.9971

6.4 Exercises

6.1 Write a WinBUGS program to estimate the overall true positive fraction using the same audiology data file as in the example above. (See Table 6.1.) Note that the cases for a true positive are not the same as those for a false positive. Estimate the effect of age, location, and severity of disease on the true positive rate with test a results only. Employ the log link function and compare your results to Table 3.9 of Pepe.[1]

6.2 Using the same dataset as in Table 6.2 for the logistic link, perform a Bayesian analysis with the log link and compare your results to Table 3.12 of Pepe.

6.3 Using the same audiology data file in Table 6.2, perform the analysis with a logistic link, but with the true positive occurrence as the dependent variable.

6.4 Using the dataset that was used in Section 6.2.2, perform a Bayesian analysis, but with the logistic link.

6.5 Devise a strategy for choosing between the log and logistic links to analyze a given set of data. Explain in detail and provide a convincing argument.

6.6 Verify the last statement about the RPDLRAB mean value of 3.696 by amending the above program to give the ratio directly. Refer to Table 6.3.

6.7 Verify the results of Table 6.5 and perform the posterior analysis for the gender specific ROC curves. Estimate the ROC areas.

6.8 To verify the results of Table 6.6, write a WinBUGS program.

6.9 Refer to Table 6.6 and Pepe(ex. 6.4, p. 144) and derive a formula for the induced ROC curve.

6.10 For the prostate cancer example, estimate the area under the ROC curve without covariates.

References

1. Pepe, M.S.,The Statistical Evaluation of Medical Tests for Classification and Prediction, Oxford University Press, 2003, Oxford, U.K.
2. Zhou, X.H., McClish, D.K., and Obuchowski, N.A., Statistical Methods in Diagnostic Medicine, John Wiley & Sons, 2002, New York.
3. Leisenring, W., Pepe, M.S., and Longton, G., A marginal regression framework for evaluating medical diagnostic tests, *Stat. Med.*, 16, 1263, 1997.
4. Leisenring, W. and Pepe, M.S., Regression modeling of diagnostic likelihood ratio tests for the evaluation of medical diagnostic tests, *Biometrics*, 54, 444, 1998.

5. Leisenring, W., Alonzo, T., and Pepe, M.S., Comparison of predictive values of binary medical diagnostic tests for paired designs, *Biometrics*, 56, 345, 2000.
6. Tosteson, A.A.N. and Begg, C.B., A general regression methodology for ROC curve estimation, *Med. Decis. Making*, 8, 204, 1988.
7. Toledano, A. and Gatsonis, C.A., Regression analysis of correlated receiver operating characteristic curves, *Acad. Radiol.*, 2, Supplement 1, S30, 1995.
8. Holtbrugge,W. and Schumacher, M., A comparison of regression models for the analysis of categorical data, *Applied Stat.*, 40, 249, 1991.
9. Gregurich, M.A., A Bayesian Approach to Estimating the Regression Coefficients of a Multinomial Logit Model, Ph.D. dissertation, The University of Texas Health Science Center at Houston, School of Public Health, 1992, Houston.
10. Etzioni, R., Pepe, M.S., Longton, G, Hu, C., and Goodman, G., Incorporating the time dimension in receiver operating characteristic curves: a case study of prostate cancer, *Med. Decis.* Making, 19, 242, 1991.

Chapter 7

Agreement

7.1 Introduction

This chapter discusses variability between readers in the diagnostic process. The readers may be radiologists, pathologists, oncologists, surgeons, etc., and it is well known that variability does indeed exist and is a problem in the medical sciences. The problem occurs because of errors in measurements due to differences in diagnoses to differences in the intrinsic accuracy of medical devices, differences in the ability and training of the radiologists or pathologists, and differences in the experimental units under study.

Shoukri[1] describes the inconsistencies and inaccuracies in various medical specialties. For example, he mentions the Birkelo et al.[2] study, which describes the variability between five readers attempting to diagnose pulmonary tuberculosis. Clinicians also exhibit much variability in routine examinations of the chest, according to Fletcher.[3] The variability between physicians in making diagnoses is common and a serious problem. The problem of inaccuracies and inconsistencies is well known in diagnostic radiology; however, the same cannot be said for other areas of medicine.

Variability between readers is a problem in clinical trials in assessing patient progress. For example, in Phase II trials, the response to therapy is often determined by a team of radiologists (among others) who classify the patient's progress based on the size of the tumor measured by a radiological device. Differences in the radiologists' assessments play an important role in the outcome of the trial. Larger differences between readers imply less confidence in the trials' conclusions. But, such variability is rarely taken into account in the conclusions of a Phase II trial. These ideas will be explored in Chapter 8.

Several studies completed at the MD Anderson Cancer Center (MDACC) on inter- and intra-observer differences between radiologists will be introduced in this chapter. They will illustrate the sources of variation and how to take them into account. These studies focus on differences between readers in the following areas: (1) in measuring the size of a liver lesions via magnetic resonance imaging (MRI) and (2) in measuring blood flow by computed tomography (CT). The analysis of agreement will focus on estimating the intra-class correlation coefficient (ICC) via the variance components of a mixed linear model. When the response is continuous, various regression techniques will be employed to measure agreement. These procedures are Bayesian analogs of the well-known frequency counterparts including the ICC and Bland–Altman methods.

The chapter starts with a description of the agreement between raters or readers when binary values are assigned by each reader to each subject (or image or specimen, etc.). This is generalized to include a discrete (more than two, but finite) number of ratings assigned by each observer to all images. Then, finally, the case of multiple observers is considered. The student will recognize this as the usual introduction to the Kappa statistic and to the McNemar test for the analysis of agreement between raters when the scores are binary. However, the approach here is strictly Bayesian. For example, for binary data, the posterior distribution of the Kappa parameter is derived. The Kappa parameter is simplified to include multiple raters, multiple ratings, and stratified situations, and is the foundation for the corresponding Bayesian analysis.

The later parts of the chapter will describe regression techniques for including patient covariate information in the analysis of agreement. The student is referred to Shoukri[1] for an introduction to the general problem of agreement, both for continuous and discrete data and to an introduction to the ICC for agreement between observers when the response is continuous.

7.2 Agreement for Discrete Ratings

7.2.1 Binary Scores

Consider the 2 × 2 in Table 7.1 that gives a binary score to n subjects. Each subject is classified as either positive or negative by both readers.

Let θ_{ij} be the probability that rater 1 gives a score of i and rater 2 a score of j, where $i, j = 0$ or 1, and let n_{ij} be the corresponding number of subjects. Obviously, the probability of agreement is the sum of the diagonal probabilities; however, this measure of agreement is usually not used. Instead, the Kappa parameter is often employed as an overall measure of agreement, and is defined as

$$\kappa = [(\theta_{00} + \theta_{11}) - (\theta_{0.}\theta_{.0} + \theta_{1.}\theta_{.1})]/[1 - (\theta_{0.}\theta_{.0} + \theta_{1.}\theta_{.1})] \tag{7.1}$$

TABLE 7.1

Classification Table

	Rater 2	
	$X = 0$	$X = 1$
Rater 1		
$X = 0$	(n_{00}, θ_{00}),	(n_{01}, θ_{01})
$X = 1$	(n_{10}, θ_{10})	(n_{11}, θ_{11})

where the dot indicates summation of the θ_{ij} over the missing subscript. Thus, the numerator of Kappa is the difference in two terms; the first is the sum of the diagonal elements and the second assumes that the raters are independent in their assignment of rating to subjects. The second term gives the probability of agreement that will occur by chance, thus Kappa is a chance corrected measure of agreement. Kappa varies over $(-\infty, 1)$ and is sometimes given the following interpretation. (See Kundel and Polansky[4] for a discussion of the interpretation of Kappa.)

Why a chance corrected index? Should there be a correction for agreement by chance? Suppose rater 1 is a radiologist using CT, while rater 2 is another radiologist aided by an MRI. Then it is reasonable to assume that the raters are using different criteria to make the positive or negative assessment of disease. If so, any agreement would be due to chance. This would not be the case if raters 1 and 2 are the same person using the same device for diagnosis and the study is one of replication testing the intra-rater consistency. In any case, the Kappa parameter can be estimated and the chance component of agreement estimated as well.

The Bayesian approach will use Minitab® to generate random samples from the posterior distribution of the θ_{ij} and, consequently, from the posterior distribution of the Kappa parameter. Once this is done, tests of hypotheses about Kappa involving the degree of agreement can be performed and sample size questions addressed.

Consider the following study of agreement with 100 cases (Table 7.2). Minitab generated 1000 samples from the joint posterior distribution of the parameters, which is Dirichlet (2,10,10,82), assuming a uniform prior distribution. Recall that this is done by first generating four independent columns with gamma variates with first-shape parameters (2,10,10,82) and a common second-shape parameter 2. The four columns are then divided by the total of the four columns, resulting in the four columns as random samples from the appropriate Dirichlet distribution. From the four columns of Dirichlet variates, the Kappa value is computed, giving 1000 samples from the posterior distribution of that parameter. The posterior analysis is shown in Table 7.3.

The posterior mean of the agreement parameter $(\theta_{00} + \theta_{11})$ and the chance agreement parameter $(\theta_{0.}\theta_{.0} + \theta_{1.}\theta_{.1})$ have almost the same posterior mean and standard deviation. This is as it should be. The table was constructed so that the readers provide independent ratings. There is a slight right

TABLE 7.2

Classification Table

	Rater 2	
	X = 0	**X = 1**
Rater 1		
X = 0	$(1, \theta_{00})$	$(9, \theta_{01})$
X = 1	$(9, \theta_{10})$	$(81, \theta_{11})$

TABLE 7.3

Posterior Distribution for Agreement

Parameter	Mean	Median	SD	95% Credible Interval
Agreement	.806	.808	.039	(.723, .875)
Chance Agreement	.794	.794	.034	(.724, .858)
Kappa	.057	.043	.032	(–.105, .297)

skewness exhibited by the posterior distribution of Kappa (Figure 7.1). For further discussion, see Fisher and Van Belle[5] (p. 527).

This example shows that there is good agreement and good chance agreement that cancel each other to give poor chance corrected agreement portrayed by the Kappa parameter. The credible interval indicates the Kappa parameter is not nonzero, which, of course, is as it should be. Since the agreement and chance agreement values are the same, Kappa should be zero. The sample size and sampling variability give empirical values that are not quite the same.

7.2.2 Other Indices of Agreement

According to Shoukri,[1] there are several other adjusted indices for agreement including the G-coefficient and the Jacquard coefficient. For more information about the former, see Maxwell.[6] The G-coefficient is defined as

$$G = [(\theta_{00} + \theta_{11}) - (\theta_{01} + \theta_{10})] \tag{7.2}$$

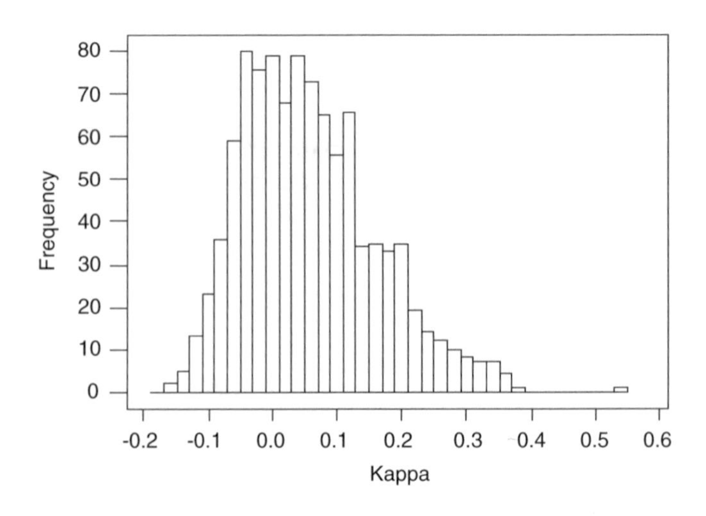

FIGURE 7.1
Posterior distribution of Kappa.

where G = 1 indicates perfect agreement and G = –1 perfect disagreement. The other measure, the Jacquard coefficient, is

$$J = \theta_{11} / (\theta_{11} + \theta_{01} + \theta_{10}), \quad 0 \le J \le 1. \tag{7.3}$$

7.2.3 A Bayesian Version of McNemar

The McNemar test examines the hypothesis that both raters have the same probability of assigning 1 to all subjects. That is

$$H: \theta_{1.} = \theta_{.1} \quad \text{vs.} \quad A: \theta_{1.} \ne \theta_{.1}. \tag{7.4}$$

Is the hypothesis rejected for the information in Table 7.2? Let $d = \theta_{1.} - \theta_{.1}$, then the histogram of 1000 values from the posterior distribution of the differences is given in Figure 7.2. The posterior mean is .0018 and the posterior standard deviation is .0437, with a 95% credible interval of (–.0857, .0872). There is little evidence that the null hypothesis is false and one concludes that both raters are using the same probability to assign the number 1 to a subject.

7.2.4 Comparing Two Kappa Parameters

Shoukri (p. 34) compares two Kappa parameters in the study of ultrasound and MRI to stage prostate cancer. The information is portrayed in Table 7.4A

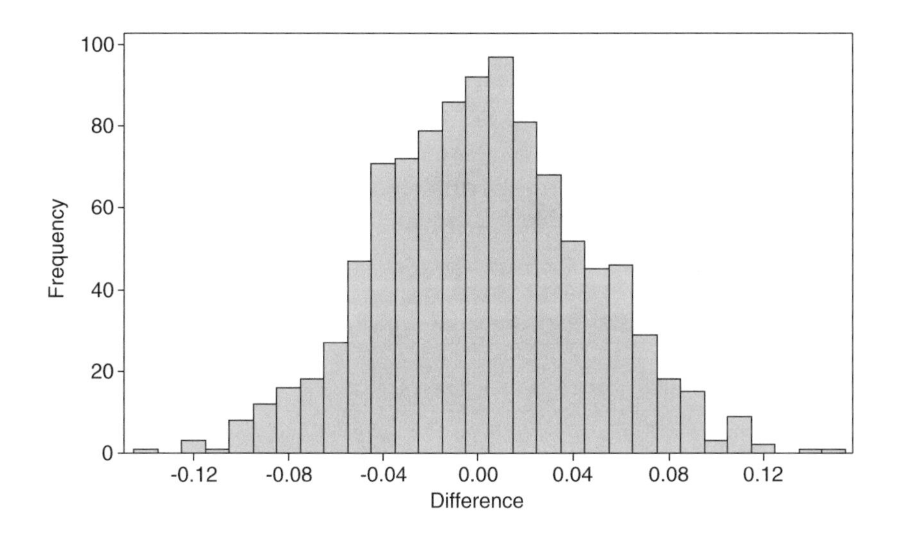

FIGURE 7.2
Posterior distribution of the difference.

TABLE 7.4A

Stageing of Prostate Cancer with Ultrasound

	Pathological Stage		
	Advanced	**Localized**	**Total**
Ultrasound Stage			
Advanced	45	50	95
Localized	60	90	150
Total	105	140	245

TABLE 7.4B

Stageing of Prostate Cancer with MRI

	Pathological Stage		
	Advanced	**Localized**	**Total**
MRI Stage			
Advanced	51	28	79
Localized	30	88	118
Total	81	116	197

and Table 7.4b. The agreement between ultrasound and pathological stage is given in the first table, while the second table presents the association between MRI and pathological staging. Pathological staging is considered the gold standard.

The comparison is based on the posterior distribution of the difference between the two Kappa parameters.

The agreement ultrasound and the agreement MRI parameters are the sum of the diagonal terms, giving the overall agreement without the adjustment for chance agreement.

It is obvious that the agreement between MRI and pathology is greater than that for ultrasound and pathology for staging prostate cancer lesions, and the 95% credible interval for the difference in the two Kappa parameters does not include zero. See Table 7.5.

TABLE 7.5

The Posterior Distributions for Comparing MRI Kappa Vs. Ultrasound Kappa

Parameter	**Mean**	**Median**	**SD**	**95% Credible Interval**
Agreement Ultra	.551	.551	.089	(.488, .611)
Chance Agreement Ultra	.515	.513	.031	(.501, .534)
Kappa Ultra	.073	.072	.008	(−.049, .196)
Agreement MRI	.704	.704	.032	(.633, .763)
Chance Agreement MRI	.517	.516	.010	(.501, .540)
Kappa MRI	.386	.386	.066	(.246, .513)
Difference = Kappa Ultra − Kappa MRI	−.312	.312	.089	(−.491, −.136)

7.2.5 Kappa and Stratification

Shourkri (p. 35), using hypothetical data, analyzes the association between MRI and ultrasound as a function of lesion size. The usual approach is to use a weighted Kappa parameter with weights chosen according to several schemes. The weighted Kappa parameter is

$$\kappa = \sum_{i=1}^{i=m} w_i \kappa_i \tag{7.5}$$

where the sum of the weights is unity, κ_i is the usual Kappa parameter for the *ith* stratum, and w_i is the weight assigned to the *ith* stratum.

There are several weighting plans, including: (1) equal weighting, (2) weighting by the sample size of a stratum, and (3) weighting by the inverse of the sampling variance of the estimated Kappa parameter. The latter two approaches appear preferable, but each has its drawbacks. For example, Barlow et al.[8] show that method (3) has smaller variance than method (2), but that it also has a larger bias.

Consider the following information on the agreement between MRI and ultrasound, stratified by lesion size and involving 300 images (Table 7.6). This information is taken from Shoukri (Table 3.6).

The analysis will use the sample size as weights for the weighted Kappa Equation (7.5). The data is grouped into three strata: the 1 to 10 mm group, the 11 to 20 mm group, and the ≥ 21 mm group, with stratum sizes of 208, 68, and 24, respectively. The posterior analysis of the three Kappa parameters is done the usual way with Minitab and 1000 generated observations from the posterior distribution. (See Section 7.2.1.) The posterior distribution of the Kappa parameter of the three strata and the overall weighted Kappa appear in Table 7.7.

TABLE 7.6

MRI and Ultrasound Stratified by Lesion Size

Lesion Size mm	Missed by Both (0,0)	Seen by MRI Only (0,1)	Seen by Ultrasound Only (1,0)	Seen by Both (1,1)	Total
1–5	40	15	10	20	85
6–10	29	14	10	70	123
11–15	10	7	7	12	36
16–20	3	2	3	24	32
21–25	0	1	1	10	12
> 25	1	2	1	8	12
Total	83	41	32	144	300

Source: Adapted from Shoukri, M.M., *Measures of Interobserver Agreement*, Chapman & Hall/ CRC, 2004, Boca Raton, FL.

TABLE 7.7

Weighted Kappa for Stratified Analysis

Parameter	Mean	Median	SD	95% Credible Interval
Kappa 1	.515	.516	.057	(.398, .621)
Kappa 2	.350	.353	.111	(.117, .575)
Kappa 3	.195	.184	.187	(–.133, .589)
Weighted Kappa	.452	.453	.049	(.350, .545)

As seen from Figure 7.3, the Kappa 3 histogram is centered to the left and the histogram of Kappa 1 to the far right, and that the variability of Kappa 1 is the largest among the three.

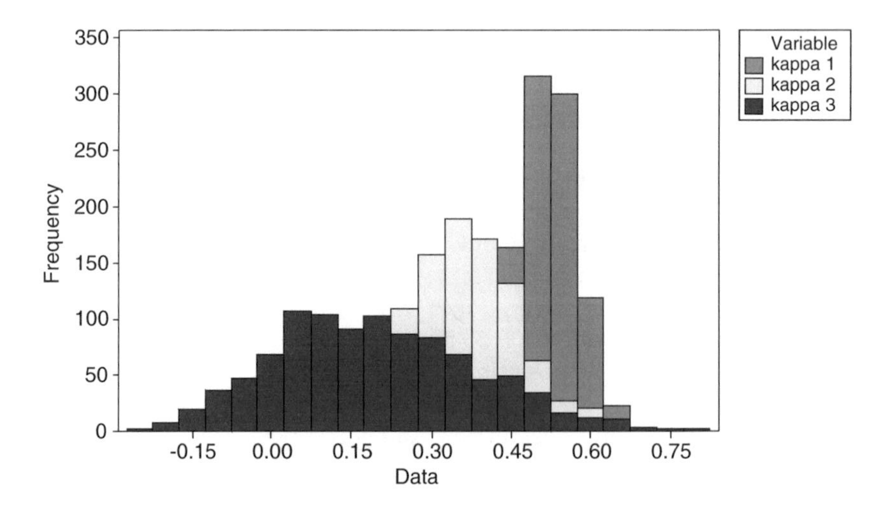

FIGURE 7.3
Posterior distribution of three Kappas.

7.2.6 Multiple Categories and Two Readers

Suppose that two radiologists are assigning c ≥ 3 discrete categories to images. How is agreement measured between the two? Kappa is generalized in an obvious way to

$$\kappa = \left[\sum_{i=1}^{i=c}(\theta_{ii} - \theta_{i.}\theta_{.i})\right] \Big/ \left[1 - \sum_{i=1}^{i=c}\theta_{i.}\theta_{.i}\right] \tag{7.6}$$

where θ_{ii} is the probability that radiologist 1 gives a score of i and radiologist 2 a score of i, where $i = 1,2,\ldots,c$. As in the binary case, the first term in the numerator is the probability of overall agreement (the sum of the probabilities

TABLE 7.8

Agreement in Diagnosis of Multiple Sclerosis between Two Neurologists

	Neurologist 2				
	1	2	3	4	Total
Neurologist 1					
1	38	5	0	1	44
2	33	11	3	0	47
3	10	14	5	6	35
4	3	7	3	10	23
Total	84	37	11	17	149

in the c × c table of joint radiologist scores), while the second term is the probability of agreement by chance. The marginal probabilities are $\theta_{i.}$ = probability that radiologist 1 gives a score of i and $\theta_{.i}$ is the probability that radiologist 2 gives a score of i. One result of more categories is that there is less chance of agreement between the two radiologists. The posterior analysis would proceed in a similar fashion as the binary case. One would have the joint Dirichlet distribution of C^2 multinomial parameters θ_{ij} and this posterior distribution is easily determined by Minitab.

Another example by Shoukri (p.44), also analyzed by Landis and Koch,[9] provides information for a Bayesian approach to estimating the agreement via Equation (7.6) between two neurologists who are diagnosing patients into one of four categories of multiple sclerosis (MS): (1) certain MS, (2) probable MS, (3) possible MS, and (4) unlikely MS. (See Table 7.8 for the outcomes.)

Thus, both neurologists diagnosed 38 patients as definitely having MS. Let θ_{ij} be the probability that neurologist 1 gives a diagnosis of i and the other a diagnosis of j where $i, j = 1, 2, 3$, and 4. Assuming a uniform prior distribution for the multinomial parameters, their posterior distribution is Dirichlet (39,6,1,2,34, 12,4,1,11,15,6,7,4,8,4,11), and the analysis is easily done with Minitab. The parameters of the Dirichlet are found by reading Table 7.8 from left to right and adding one to each cell entry. The posterior distribution is based on 1000 observations generated from the above distribution and as shown in Table 7.9.

The posterior distribution for the overall agreement is .412, but when adjusted for chance, Kappa is estimated as .188 with the median. Kappa

TABLE 7.9

Posterior Distribution of Kappa for Agreement of Neurologists

Parameter	Mean	SD	Median	95% Credible Interval
Overall Agreement	.413	.037	.412	
Agreement by Chance	.275	.014	.273	
Kappa	.191	.047	.188	(.103, .289)

appears to be nonzero and is also estimated by the 95% credible interval (.103, .289), thus giving poor to fair agreement in the diagnosis of MS between the two neurologists.

7.2.7 Multiple Categories

Shoukri (p. 50) presents the diagnoses of cervical vertebral malformation made by four veterinarian students. They were presented with 20 X-ray images with the following binary ratings, where 0 indicates no malformation and 1 designates malformation (Table 7.10).

Two X-rays received the ratings 0, 0, 0, and 0 by students 1, 2, 3, and 4, respectively. Also, no X-ray received the ratings 0, 0, 0, and 1.

Let θ_{ijkl} be the probability that students 1, 2, 3, and 4 give ratings i, j, k, and l, respectively, to an X-ray, where $i, j, k, l = 0, 1$. Then the θ_{ijkl} have a Dirichlet distribution and, via Minitab, samples are easily generated from the joint distribution. How is agreement measured with four readers? A Kappa parameter can be estimated for the agreement of all four students.

The probability that all four agree is $ag = (\theta_{0000} + \theta_{1111})$ and the probability all agreeing by chance is

$$agc = [(\theta_{0...} * \theta_{.0..} * \theta_{..0.} * \theta_{...0}) + (\theta_{1...} * \theta_{.1..} * \theta_{..1.} * \theta_{...1})],$$

where $\theta_{i...}$ is the probability that student 1 gives a rating of i, $i = 0, 1$, etc. If the four students are assigning scores independently, $\theta_{0000} = (\theta_{0...} * \theta_{.0..} * \theta_{..0.} * \theta_{...0})$, etc.

Thus, Kappa is

$$\kappa = (\text{ag} - \text{agc})/(1 - \text{agc}). \tag{7.7}$$

TABLE 7.10

Ratings of 20 X-Rays by 4 Students

Rating	Frequency
0 0 0 0	2
0 0 0 1	0
0 0 1 0	2
0 1 0 0	0
1 0 0 0	3
1 1 1 0	0
1 1 0 1	2
1 0 1 1	1
0 1 1 1	0
0 0 1 1	0
0 1 0 1	1
1 0 0 1	0
0 1 1 0	0
1 1 0 0	1
1 0 1 0	1
1 1 1 1	7
Total	20

The G-coefficient for total agreement is

$$G = (ag - (1 - ag)) \tag{7.8}$$

and is adjusted for the probability of nonagreement.

On the other hand, because there are multiple raters, partial agreement is possible. For example, what is the probability that at least three students agree? It is

$$ag3 = ag + (\theta_{0001} + \theta_{0010} + \theta_{0100} + \theta_{1000} + \theta_{1110} + \theta_{1101} + \theta_{1011} + \theta_{0111}). \tag{7.9}$$

When considering partial agreement, it is convenient to use a G-type coefficient, namely

$$G_3 = (ag3 - (1 - ag3)). \tag{7.10}$$

What are the posterior distributions of these measures of total and partial agreement? (See Table 7.11.)

Total agreement of all four students is quite poor, estimated by the Kappa parameter as .163 and a credible interval that includes 0. Also, the G-coefficient is negative, indicating poor total agreement, but the partial agreement of at least three students is judged as fairly good, with a G-coefficient of .640 (the maximum value is 1).

TABLE 7.11

Posterior Distribution of Total and Partial Agreement of Four Students

Parameter	Mean	Median	SD	95% Credible Interval
ag, total agreement of four students	.332	.331	.082	
agc, agreement by chance of all four	.198	.183	.058	
Kappa, for agreement of all four students	.163	.170	.117	(–.067, .369)
G-coefficient for total agreement of all four students	–.334	–.336	.164	(–.648, –.005)
*ag*3, agreement of at least three students	.819	.820	.096	
G_3, G-coefficient for agreement of at least three students	.639	.640	.193	(.264, 1.000)

7.2.8 Agreement and Covariate Information

How is patient covariate information included in the measure of agreement between radiologists? Consider the G-coefficient defined as

$$G = [(\theta_{00} + \theta_{11}) - (\theta_{01} + \theta_{10})], \tag{7.2}$$

for the 2 × 2 classification in Table 7.1. Note that agreement occurs with probability

$$ag = (\theta_{00} + \theta_{11}) \quad (7.11)$$

and that of nonagreement with probability

$$nag = 1 - ag = (\theta_{01} + \theta_{10}). \quad (7.12)$$

Since the occurrence of agreement is scored as a binary event, it is natural to use logistic regression in order to determine the effect of covariates on ag and, thus, on the G-coefficient. Therefore, let

$$G(x) = \{ag(x) - [1 - ag(x)]\} = 2ag(x) - 1 \quad (7.13)$$

and consider the example of stratification in Table 7.6. However, suppose the lesion size of each patient is used as the covariate x in $G(x)$. Logistic regression is used to regress the logit of $ag(x)$ on x where x is the lesion size of a patient.

There are 300 patients and on each the lesions size is assigned as in Table 7.12. Refer to Table 7.6 where there are six categories of lesion size and four categories of the joint classification of MRI and ultrasound.

A random sample of 70 lesion sizes is selected from the discrete uniform distribution (6,7,8,9,10) and assigned to the 70 patients.

A logistic regression is performed where the dependent variable is the occurrence of agreement between MRI and ultrasound. Agreement occurs when a patient is missed (0,0) by both modalities or seen (1,1) by both. The logistic model is

$$\text{Logit}[ag(x)/(1 - ag(x))] = \beta_1 + \beta_2 * x \quad (7.14)$$

TABLE 7.12

Lesion Size for Agreement of MRI and Ultrasound

Lesion Size mm	Missed by Both (0,0)	Seen by MRI Only (0,1)	Seen by Ultrasound Only (1,0)	Seen by Both (1,1)	Total
1–5	40: 1–2	15: 2–3	10: 23	20: 3–5	85
6–10	29: 6–7	14: 7–8	10: 7–8	70: 6–10*	123
11–15	10: 11–12	7: 12–13	7: 12–13	12: 13–15	36
16–20	3: 16–17	2: 17–18	3: 17–18	24: 18–20	32
21–25	0: 21–22	1: 22–23	1: 22–23	10: 23–25	12
> 26	1: 26–30	2: 28–31	1: 28–31	8: 31-35	12
Total	83	41	32	144	300

where x is the lesion size. The following program is executed to estimate the beta parameters.

```
model
{


# x1 is lesion size
#x2 is agreement
for( i in 1 : 300 ) {
x2[i] ~ dbern(p[i])
logit(p[i]) <- beta[1] + beta[2] * x1[i]
q[i]<- exp(beta[1]+beta[2]*x1[i])/
(1+exp(1+beta[1]+beta[2]*x1[i]))
}
phat<-mean(p[])
qhat <- mean(q[])
for (i in 1:2 ){
beta[i] ~ dnorm(0.0,0.0001)}
}
```

The dependent vector is ×2[] and gives the occurrence of agreement, while the vector of 300 lesion sizes is denoted by ×1[]. The posterior analysis for the beta coefficients is given in Table 7.13.

Thus, the G-coefficient depends on x where

$$G(x) = 2ag(x) - 1$$

and

$$ag(x) = \exp(.893 + .026x)/[1 + \exp(.893 + .026x)]. \tag{7.15}$$

Note that $ag(x)$ is the probability of agreement when the lesion size is x. For this example, the effect of lesion size is minimal. Of course, in practice, the covariate is often stratified and the G-coefficient estimated in each stratum, and then a weighted G-coefficient is formed for an overall estimate of agreement.

TABLE 7.13

Logistic Regression for Agreement: Effect of Lesion Size

Parameter	Mean	Median	SD	95% Credible Interval
Beta[1]	.893	.890	.224	(.453, 1.336)
Beta[2]	.026	.026	.019	(–.011, .067)

7.3 Agreement for a Continuous Response

7.3.1 Introduction

What does it take for two raters to agree? If the two produce identical paired values on the same units, then they agree perfectly, and everyone would agree on this definition. Of course, this is not seen very often. There are many ways for raters to agree. For example, the average of their paired responses could be the same or the standard deviations of the responses could be similar. The correlation between the two paired responses could be high. Or, if one reader's response is regressed on the other's response, the fitted line could go through the origin with slope 1. The correlation between readers can be high, but their mean values can be far apart. Thus, agreement is a multifaceted phenomenon, in that two readers may agree according to one criterion, but not agree with respect to another.

Readers do not agree, however, because of the randomness inherent in the study. The randomness in the raters' responses is caused by a variety of sources including differences in the experimental units, differences between the ability and experience of the raters, and differences in the measuring devices (e.g., MRI, ultrasound, nuclear medicine techniques for diagnostic radiology, or the differences in the histology methods of pathologists).

This requires statistical methods to assess the degree of agreement. The basic descriptive statistics should always be computed, namely the mean, median, and standard deviation, listed by reader and, if necessary, by replications within readers. This should be accompanied by graphical methods including Box plots (tools that display centering, spread, and distribution of a continuous dataset) of the various responses, again listed by reader and replication. This will give the inter- and intra-observer variation. The descriptive statistics by themselves can tell almost the whole story about the agreement between readers.

Based on the descriptive statistics and the graphical evidence, specialized procedures can be invoked in order to further explore agreement. For continuous variables, regression and analysis of variance methods are the most appropriate. For example, using the one-way random model where the levels of the main factor are the different images of the study, and where the readers are considered random, the intra-class correlation coefficient (ICC) estimates the correlation between two readers within images. The ICC approach is also appropriate for two-way layouts when there is replication of a reader's scores. Another use of the random model is to partition the total variance into the sum of the variances of the various factors in the model. Suppose there are three readers with replicate readings of the same image, then there are several sources of variation, including patients, readers, replications (within readers), and error. Each factor will have an associated variance component, which is estimated by a Bayesian procedure. The sum of the four variance components is the total variance of the experiment, thus the percent of the total variation due to each source can be estimated. It has been the author's experience that the between patient variance component is always dominant and that the component for the replication factor is the smallest. These ideas will be illustrated with an example from MDACC.

Linear regression methods may also be employed to assess the degree of agreement between two readers. For example, suppose two readers are measuring lesion size on the same set of images, so that their responses are paired. The lesion size of one reader is regressed on the lesion size of other and the intercept and slope estimated. If the two are in agreement, one would expect the intercept to be zero and the slope to be 1. Indeed, if the two were in perfect agreement, their paired values would be identical and the fitted line would go through the origin with a slope of 1. On the other hand, if the fitted line is far from going through the origin and/or, if the estimated slope is not close to 1, this is evidence that the two readers are not in agreement. Bayesian regression techniques will be employed to assess agreement. Additional regression methods for agreement include the Bland–Altman procedure, but will not be pursued here. A good introduction to agreement with continuous data is in Fleiss[10] (Chap. 1). Shoukri[1] is also a good, wide-ranging reference to the general subject of agreement, including the use of mixed and random models for estimating the ICC.

7.3.2 Intra-class Correlation Coefficient

7.3.2.1 One-Way Random Model

Let y_{ij} denote the observation in the *ith* row and *jth* column where

$$y_{ij} = \theta_i + e_{ij} \tag{7.16}$$

where the $\theta_i \sim nid(\theta, \sigma_b^2)$ are independent of the $e_{ij} \sim nid(0, \sigma_w^2)$, for $i = 1,2,\ldots,r$ and $j = 1,2,\ldots,c$. The intra-class correlation coefficient is

$$\rho = \sigma_b^2 / \left(\sigma_b^2 + \sigma_w^2\right) \tag{7.17}$$

and is the correlation between the two distinct observations in the same row. Note that if $j \neq j'$

$$\begin{aligned} \mathrm{cov}(y_{ij}, y_{ij'}) &= \mathrm{cov}(\theta_i + e_{ij}, \theta_i + e_{ij'}) \\ &= \mathrm{cov}(\theta_i, \theta_i) = \sigma_b^2 \end{aligned} \tag{7.18}$$

and the ICC of Equation (7.17) is confirmed.

In diagnostic radiology, the rows usually represent images and the columns readers, thus ICC is the common correlation between the ratings of pairs of the reader.

TABLE 7.14

Descriptive Statistics of Lesion Size by Reader

Reader	Mean (mm)	Median	SD	Interquartile Range
1	37.21	34.34	26.01	26.00
2	32.75	26.50	18.54	30.75
3	33.57	27.00	24.47	32.00

Recently Kundra[11] conducted a study involving the comparison of six MRI sequences for the diagnosis of liver lesions. Three readers and 22 patients were involved and the readers read the same image twice. There were multiple lesions in the liver and, as part of the study, the lesion size of the "largest" lesion was measured. This was done by measuring the major axis of the lesion. The descriptive statistics are displayed in Table 7.14.

The Box plots of Figure 7.4 show the inter-reader variation in measuring the major axis of the largest lesion of 22 patients, who were imaged with the fast spin echo sequence. The plots reveal that readers 2 and 3 are in good agreement with regard to the median lesion size and that they also have similar variations about the median, as measured by the interquartile range.

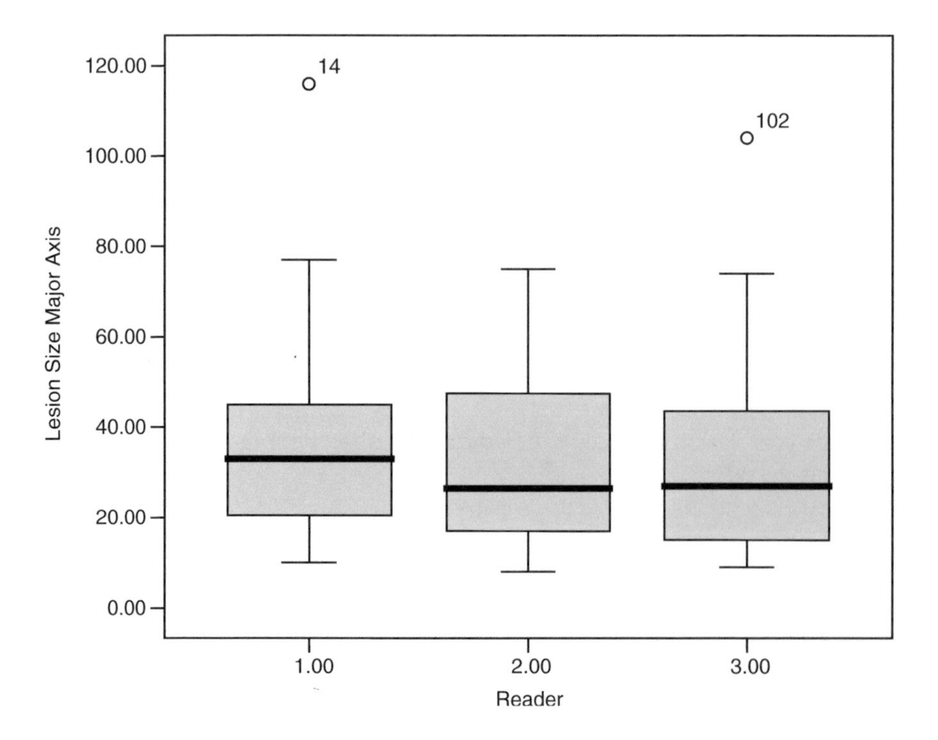

FIGURE 7.4
Box plots of inter-reader variation for lesion size.

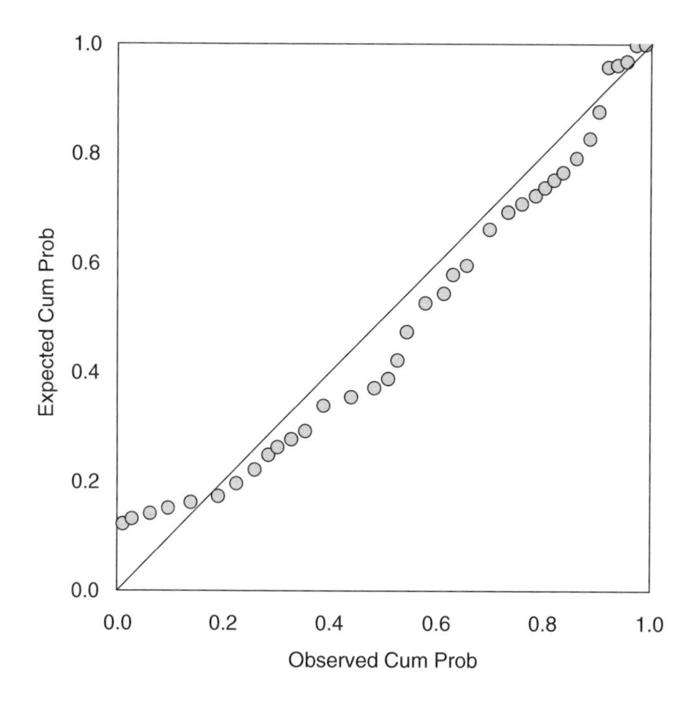

FIGURE 7.5
P-P plot of lesion size.

Also, shown in Figure 7.5, is a P-P plot to assess the goodness of the fit of the 22 lesion values for reader 1. This test for normality shows that the values do not depart too much from the assumption of normality, a preliminary test that is necessary for the analysis via the random one-way model.

Table 7.15 provides the posterior analysis for estimating the intra-class correlation coefficient Equation (7.17). For this example, only one replication for each reader is included and only one MRI sequence (fast spin echo) was considered. The program does give all the necessary information and the data are included. The between and within variance components are denoted by sigma2.b and sigma2.w, and the y matrix in the data list is the 22×3 matrix of lesion size values. The NA denotes a missing value.

TABLE 7.15
Posterior Distribution of the Intra-Class Correlation Coefficient

Parameter	Mean	Median	SD	95% Credible Interval
ρ	.793	.793	.071	(.624, .903)
σ_b^2	444.7	413	166	(219.4, 851.6)
σ_w^2	108.8	104.6	27.4	(67.93, 174)
θ	33.24	33.24	4.72	(23.9, 42.57)

```
model
{
for( i in 1 : patients ) {
m[i] ~ dnorm(theta, tau.b)
for( j in 1 : readers ) {
y[i , j] ~ dnorm(m[i], tau.w)
}
}
sigma2.w <- 1 / tau.w
sigma2.b <- 1 / tau.b
tau.w ~ dgamma(0.001, 0.001)
tau.b ~ dgamma(0.001, 0.001)
theta ~ dnorm(0.0, 1.0E-10)
ICC<-sigma2.b/(sigma2.b+sigma2.w)
}
list(patients = 22, readers = 3,
y = structure(.Data = c( 26.00, 22.00, 10.00,
NA, 25.00, 25.00,
NA, NA, 10.00,
NA, 17.00, 19.00,
20.00, 17.00, NA,
30.00, 28.00, NA,
39.00, 44.00, 40.00,
33.00, 53.00, 40.00,
46.00, 47.00, 27.00,
26.00, 25.00, 26.00,
50.00, 51.00, 49.00,
44.00, 48.00, 47.00,
77.00, 75.00, 74.00,
116.00, 44.00, 104.00,
11.00, 8.00, 12.00,
10.00, 12.00, 9.00,
12.00, 12.00, 15.00,
61.00, 56.00, 53.00,
21.00, 21.00, 27.00,
13.00, 13.00, 15.00,
```

```
36.00, NA,NA,
36.00, 37.00, 36.00), .Dim = c(22, 3)))
list(theta= 34.48 ,tau.w=1, tau.b=1)
```

Therefore, the intra-class correlation coefficient is estimated as .79 with a 95% credible interval of (.624, .903) indicating fairly good agreement between the three readers. The analysis was based on 100,000 observations generated from the joint posterior distribution of the model parameters. The theta parameter is the overall mean with a credible interval of (23.9, 42.57). Figure 7.6 illustrates the graph of the posterior density of the ICC.

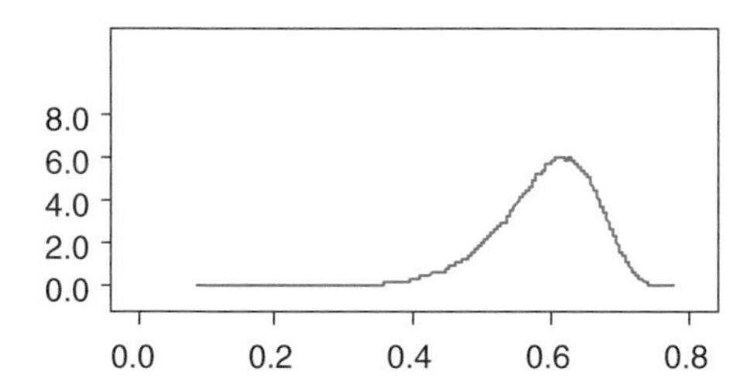

FIGURE 7.6
Posterior density of ρ.

7.3.2.2 Two-Way Random Model

Let

$$y_{ijk} = \lambda + \theta_i + \phi_j + e_{ijk} \tag{7.19}$$

where $\lambda \sim n(\mu, \sigma_\lambda^2)$, the $\theta_i \sim nid(0, \sigma_\theta^2)$, the $\phi_j \sim nid(0, \sigma_\phi^2)$, and the $e_{ijk} \sim nid\ (0, \sigma^2)$, where $i = 1,2,\ldots,r$, $j = 1,2,\ldots,c$, and $k = 1,2,\ldots,n$.

This is a two-way random model with two major factors. For our use, r is the number of images, c the number of radiologists, and n the number of replications, that is, each radiologist reads each image n times. With regard to the MRI study of the previous section, $r = 22$ lesions, $c = 3$ radiologists, and $n = 2$ replications. With this model, the intra-observer variability can be measured by

$$\rho_{intra} = corr(y_{ijk}, y_{ijk'}), \quad k \neq k'$$

$$= \left(\sigma_\lambda^2 + \sigma_\theta^2 + \sigma_\phi^2\right) / \left(\sigma_\lambda^2 + \sigma_\theta^2 + \sigma_\phi^2 + \sigma^2\right). \tag{7.20}$$

In a similar manner, the inter-observer variability may be measured by

$$\rho_{inter} = corr(y_{ijk}, y_{ij'k}), \quad j \neq j'. \tag{7.21}$$

7.3.3 Regression and Agreement

There are several regression techniques for agreement between readers providing continuous scores for diagnosis. The previous study of Kundra[11] provides a nice illustration from diagnostic radiology where there were 3 radiologists measuring the lesion size of liver lesions in 22 patients. The design was balanced and the readers were matched with the images and each radiologist read each image twice. Also, there were six imaging modalities, corresponding to six MRI sequences. A MRI sequence is a particular setting for controlling the way the magnetic field is perturbed by the radio signal, thus six different images of the same lesion are produced. The various sequences display different image qualities. A small subset of the Kundra study is employed for the use of Bayesian regression method.

If two readers agree perfectly, they would have identical readings for lesion size for the same image and the graph of one reader's readings on the other reader's would look like a line that passes closest to the origin with a slope of approximately 1. Thus, the approach is to use linear regression by regressing the scores of one reader on the scores of the other. For example, Kundra considers 22 lesion size values for readers 1 and 2 on the first replication using the first MRI sequence (fast spin echo). Regress reader 1 scores on reader 2 scores with the following program.

```
model;
{
# likelihood function
for(i in 1:N) {

y[i]~ dnorm(mu[i], precy);
mu[i] <- beta[1] + beta[2]*x[i];
}
# prior distributions - noninformative prior; similarly
for informative priors
for(i in 1:P) {
beta[i] ~ dnorm(0, 0.000001);
}
precy~dgamma(.00001,.00001)
sigma<-1/precy
}
```

```
list( N = 22, P = 2, y = c(26.00,NA,NA,NA,20.00,30.00,
39.00,33.00,46.00,26.00,50.00,
44.00,77.00,116.00,11.00,10.00,
12.00,61.00,21.00,13.00,36.00,
36.00),
x = c(22.00,25.00,24,17.00,17.00,28.00,
44.00,53.00,47.00,25.00,51.00,48.00,
75.00,44.00,8.00,12.00,12.00,56.00,
21.00,13.00,35,37.00))
list( beta = c(0,0), precy = 1 )
```

TABLE 7.16

Posterior Distribution of the Intercept and Slope: Regression of Reader 1 on Reader 2 Lesion Size

Parameter	Mean	Median	SD	95% Credible Interval
Intercept beta[1]	1.804	1.78	9.24	(–6.53, 20.31)
Slope beta[2]	1.038	1.03	.24	(.561, 1.518)
Standard deviation about regression line	366.3	337.2	140.9	(181.6, 725.5)

Based on the 95% credible intervals of Table 7.16, the slope is 1 and the intercept is zero, indicting good agreement between readers 1 and 2. The graph of Figure 7.7 confirms these informal statements. Of course, for a

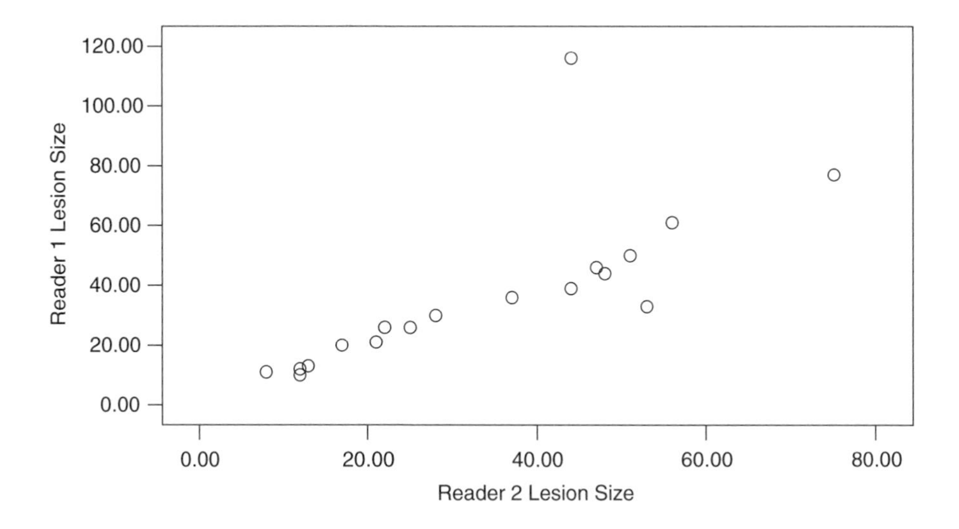

FIGURE 7.7
Reader 1 vs. reader 2.

complete analysis, the procedure should be repeated for all pairs of readers for each replication.

7.4 Combining Reader Information

Returning to the example of Kundra[11] where there were three readers estimating the size of liver lesions, suppose this information is used to judge the efficacy of treatment in a clinical trial. The change in lesion size is estimated by comparing the subsequent readings of lesion size to the baseline readings and classifying the response into one of several categories, including complete response, partial response, stable disease, or progressive disease. Which category a patient is assigned to depends on the percent change from baseline. This will be looked at in detail in the following chapter.

In such a scenario, often two readers are used to estimate the size of a lesion on each image, but if they disagree, the third radiologist adjudicates the disagreement. Another approach will be pursued here: A statistical alternative where the reader information is averaged over all the readers. How is this done from a Bayesian approach?

Assuming the lesion sizes are normally distributed, the three scores from the readers on the same image could be considered a random sample of size 22 (there are 22 patients, one lesion per patient) from a three-dimensional multivariate normal distribution. If vague prior information is employed, the posterior distribution of the mean image size has a multivariate t-distribution with 19 degrees of freedom, mean vector

$$\bar{x} = \begin{pmatrix} 37.21 \\ 32.75 \\ 33.57 \end{pmatrix} \tag{7.22}$$

and precision matrix

$$T = n(n-k)S^{-1} \tag{7.23}$$

where n is the sample size ($n = 22$ patients), k = number of measurements ($k = 3$), the number of radiologists, and S is the 3×3 sum of squares and cross products matrix, thus, the matrix of sample variances and covariances is $S/(n-k)$. In this case

$$S = \begin{pmatrix} 676.52, & 14.06, & 18.31 \\ 14.06, & 343.73, & 14.32 \\ 18.31, & 14.32, & 598.78 \end{pmatrix} \tag{7.24}$$

and

$$\theta \sim t_3(n-k, \bar{x}, n(n-k)S^{-1}). \tag{7.25}$$

Note that

$$E(\theta) = \bar{x}. \tag{7.26}$$

The dispersion matrix is

$$D(\theta) = S/[n(n-k-s)]. \tag{7.27}$$

For more information on the multivariate t-distribution, see DeGroot[12] (Chap. 5) and Box and Tiao[13] (Chap. 8).

The vague prior density for the multivariate normal is

$$f(\theta, T) \propto 1/|T|^{(k+1)/2}.$$

Of particular importance is the information on the marginal distribution of the components of θ. The marginal distribution on, say, the first component is

$$\theta_1 \sim t(n-k, \bar{x}_1, T_{11} - T_{22}T_{21}) \tag{7.28}$$

where T_{11} is scalar and consists of the element in the first row and first column of the precision matrix T, Equation (7.23), T_{12} is the row consisting of the second and third elements of the first row of T, T_{21} is the transpose of T_{21}, and T_{22} is the 2×2 matrix consisting of the lower righthand corner of T.

Having determined the posterior distribution of θ, how is the information from the three readers averaged to give an overall estimate of lesion size? One approach is to use a weighted average where each reader's mean is weighted by the inverse of the variance of the posterior distribution for the reader's mean. For example, the posterior mean of the first reader is 37.21 cm and is weighted by the inverse of the posterior distribution of θ_1. Of course, from Equation (7.23) and Equation (7.28), the precision of θ_1 is easily determined. The weighted mean is

$$\bar{\theta} = \sum_{i=1}^{i=3} E(\theta_i / data) w_i \tag{7.29}$$

where $w_i = \text{var}^{-1}(\theta_i / data) / \Sigma_{i=1}^{i=3} \text{var}^{-1}(\theta_i / data)$. The mean and variance of the posterior distribution of θ_i is $E(\theta_i / data)$ and $\text{var}(\theta_i / data)$, respectively.

7.5 Exercises

7.1 Perform the "classical" estimation of Kappa and give a 95% confidence interval for Kappa; compare to the Bayesian analysis reported in Table 7.3.

7.2 Discuss the advantages and disadvantages of G and J as measures of agreement and compare them to the Kappa parameter, and find the posterior distribution of G and J based on the information in Table 7.2.

7.3 Test the sharp null hypothesis H vs. the alternative A in Section 7.2.3 using the formal test procedure outlined in Chapter 4, Section 4.5.3.3, for comparing two binomial populations. Assume the prior probability of the null hypothesis is .5 and that, under the alternative hypothesis, the prior distribution of the two binomial parameters are independent and uniform over (0,1).

7.4 Perform the "classical" McNemar test from the information in Table 7.2 and compare to the Bayesian test in the previous exercise.

7.5 Compute Pr(Kappa MRI > Kappa Ultra/data). Use the information in Table 7.4A and Table 7.4B. Does this probability complement the conclusions in Table 7.5?

7.6 From Table 7.7, perform a weighted Kappa analysis, but use the inverse of the posterior variance as the stratum weight and compare your Kappa with the weighted Kappa in the table. Which one has the smaller posterior variance? Test the null hypothesis that your weighted Kappa is less than .36 vs. the alternative that is at least .36. State and justify your conclusions.

7.7 In Table 7.6, quadruple the sample sizes and assess the effect on the standard deviation of the weighted Kappa, using the strata sample sizes as weights. Is the standard deviation of the "new" weighted Kappa smaller than that of the weighted Kappa in the table?

7.8 Estimate the G-coefficient for partial agreement of at least two students. Use Minitab and perform the posterior analysis, similar to that given in Table 7.11.

7.9 (a) Use the above program to find an average value of agreement between MRI and ultrasound. (b) Also stratify on x to give the 6 strata of Table 7.12 and estimate the G-coefficient in each stratum, then form an overall weighted G-coefficient. Compare the weighted G-coefficient with the average value of agreement in part (a).

7.10 Derive a formula for the inter-observer variability (Equation (7.21)) in terms of a ratio of sum of variance components similar to Equation (7.20).

7.11 Based on the program of Section 7.3.2.1, write a similar program to find the posterior distribution for the intra- and inter-observer variability. The dataset is given herein.

```
list( y = structure(.Data = c(
 26.00,   38.00,   22.00,   48.00,   10.00,    NA,
 NA,      NA,      25.00,   26.00,   25.00,    25.00,
 NA,      NA,      NA,      NA,      10.00,    12.00,
 NA,      20.00,   17.00,   17.00,   19.00,    18.00,
 20.00,   21.00,   17.00,   14.00,   NA,       NA,
 30.00,   31.00,   28.00,   28.00,   NA,       30.00,
 39.00,   38.00,   44.00,   43.00,   40.00,    39.00,
 33.00,   33.00,   53.00,   39.00,   40.00,    35.00,
 46.00,   44.00,   47.00,   54.00,   27.00,    27.00,
 26.00,   27.00,   25.00,   NA,      26.00,    27.00,
 50.00,   48.00,   51.00,   45.00,   49.00,    48.00,
 44.00,   43.00,   48.00,   41.00,   47.00,    47.00,
 77.00,   79.00,   75.00,   70.00,   74.00,    73.00,
 116.00,  101.00,  44.00,   43.00,   104.00,   88.00,
 11.00,   NA,      8.00,    NA,      12.00,    NA,
 10.00,   11.00,   12.00,   14.00,   9.00,     9.00,
 12.00,   10.00,   12.00,   12.00,   15.00,    13.00,
 61.00,   65.00,   56.00,   65.00,   53.00,    61.00,
 21.00,   21.00,   21.00,   30.00,   27.00,    22.00,
 13.00,   14.00,   13.00,   15.00,   15.00,    15.00,
 36.00,   NA,      NA,      NA,      NA,       NA,
 36.00,   35.00,   37.00,   37.00,   36.00,    33.00), .Dim = c(22, 3, 2)))
```

y is a matrix with dimension $22 \times 3 \times 2$, indexed as $i = 1,2,\ldots,22$, $j = 1,2,3$, and $k = 1,2$, for the 22 lesions, 3 radiologists, and 2 replications.

7.12 Define a random model that includes patients, readers, reps, and modalities as the main factors and derive a formula similar to Equation (7.20) for the parameter that measures the intra-observer variation.

7.13 The unweighted Kappa parameter (Equation (7.6)) is appropriate when the diagnostic categories are nominal; that is, the categories are not ordinal. Are the MS categories ordinal? For ordinal scores, Cohen[14] introduced the weighted Kappa parameter

$$\kappa_w = \left[\sum_{i=1}^{i=c}\sum_{j=1}^{j=c} w_{ij}(\theta_{ij} - \theta_{i.}\theta_{.j})\right] \Bigg/ \left[1 - \sum_{i=1}^{i=c}\sum_{j=1}^{j=c} w_{ij}\theta_{i.}\theta_{.j}\right]. \tag{7.7}$$

Estimate the agreement (Equation (7.7)) between the two radiologists of Table 7.7 using assigned weights $w_{ij} = 1-(i-j)^2/(c-1)^2$, and compare to the estimated unweighted Kappa of Table 7.7. Which is the more reliable estimator?

7.14 Find the posterior distribution of the G-coefficient when the lesion size is $x = 15$ mm, and estimate the agreement between MRI and ultrasound. See Equation (7.15).

7.15 Refer to the example given in Section 7.4, using the Kundra[11] data. Compute the weighted average of the lesion size by weighting the mean of the posterior distribution of a reader's mean by the inverse of the variance of the posterior distribution of the reader's mean. That is, weight the posterior mean of θ_i by the inverse of the variance of the posterior distribution of θ_i. See Equation (7.29).

7.16 Refer to Section 7.4. Assuming that the mean vector and precision matrix of the multivariate normal are unknown, what is the conjugate prior density of θ and T?

7.17 Gayed[15] performed a cardiac perfusion study using MRI to measure cardiac function in cancer patients. One measure of cardiac function is the amount of ischemia in the cardiac wall. Two determinations of ischemia were made: one by multiple readers and the other by an independent blinded radiologist. (See Table 7.17.)

(a) Assuming a uniform prior and using formula (7.6), find the posterior distribution of Kappa.

(b) Find the posterior distribution of the G-coefficient as defined for multiple categories.

(c) What is the usual Kappa value and how does it compare to the Bayesian estimates of the Kappa parameter?

TABLE 7.17

MRI Results: Problem 17

	Blinded Reader			
	Ischemia	**Scarring**	**Normal**	**Total**
Multiple Readers				
Ischemia	12	0	1	13
Scarring	0	3	2	5
Normal	1	0	33	34
Total	13	3	36	52

18. Gayed also studied the agreement between multiple readers and one blinded reader for scoring wall motion of the heart. The ratings for wall motion are normal, moderate, mild, and marked and are given in Table 7.18.

(a) Assuming a uniform prior distribution, find the usual Kappa value for agreement in wall motion scores.

(b) What is the posterior distribution of the Kappa parameter and the G-coefficient?

(c) Which of the two is preferred?

TABLE 7.18

MRI Agreement: Problem 18

	Blinded Reader				
	Normal	**Moderate**	**Mild**	**Marked**	**Total**
Multiple Readers					
Normal	38	0	4	0	42
Moderate	0	1	0	0	1
Mild	3	0	3	0	6
Marked	0	0	0	2	2
Total	41	1	7	2	51

References

1. Shoukri, M.M., *Measures of Inter Observer Agreement*, Chapman & Hall/CRC, 2004, Boca Raton, FL.
2. Birkelo, C.C., Chamberlin, W.E., Phelps, P.S., Schools, P.E., Zacks, D., and Yerushalmy, Tuberculosis case finding – a comparison of effectiveness of various roentgenographic and photoflurographic methods, *J. Am. Med. Assoc.*, 133, 359, 1947.
3. Fletcher, C.M., The clinical diagnosis of clinical emphysema: an experimental study, *Proc. Roy. Soc. Med.*, 45, 577, 1952.
4. Kundel, H.L. and Polansky, M., Measurement of observer agreement, *Radiology*, 228, 303, 2003.
5. Fisher, L.D. and Van Belle, G., *Biostatistics: A Methodology for the Health Sciences*, John Wiley & Sons, 1993, New York.
6. Maxwell, A.E., Coefficient of agreement between observers and their interpretation, *Br. J. Psych.*, 130, 79, 1977.
7. McNemar, Q., A note on the sampling error of the difference between correlated proportions or percentages, *Psychometrika*, 12, 153, 1947.
8. Barlow, W., Lai, M.Y., and Azen, S.P., A comparison of methods forcalculating a stratified Kappa, *Stat. Med.*, 10, 1465, 1991.
9. Landis, J.R. and Koch, G.G., The measurement of observer agreement for categorical data, *Biometrics*, 33, 159, 1977.
10. Fleiss, J.L., *The Design and Analysis of Clinical Experiments*, John Wiley & Sons, 1986, New York.
11. Kundra, V., Personal Communication, 2006.
12. DeGroot, M.H., *Optimal Statistical Decisions*, McGraw-Hill, 1970, New York.
13. Box, G.E.P. and Tiao, G.C., *Bayesian Inference in Statistical Analysis*, Addison Wesley, 1973, Reading, MA.
14. Cohen, J., Weighted Kappa, nominal scale agreement with provision for scaled disagreement or partial credit, *Psychol. Bull.*,70, 213, 1968.
15. Gayed, I., Personal Communication, 2006.

Chapter 8

Diagnostic Imaging and Clinical Trials

8.1 Introduction

This chapter describes the interplay between diagnostic procedures and therapeutic clinical trials. Indeed, diagnostic imaging is a crucial element in the design and conduct of most clinical trials in oncology. For example, diagnostic imaging is present in Phase I trials for safety studies of new therapies, be they chemotherapy, radiotherapy, or biological. In order to monitor the safety and efficacy endpoints of such trials, imaging procedures determine the advance and extent of the disease and produce the primary and secondary endpoints. The chapter introduces the three phases of clinical trials and how imaging plays a role in the conduct of each trial. This is followed by a description of the protocol for clinical trials in oncology and a brief description of the protocol review process at the MD Anderson Cancer Center (MDACC). The RECIST (response evaluation criteria in solid tumors) criteria for response to therapy are introduced. This is a set of guidelines for the radiologists in their determination of the patient's response to therapy and, hence, on the conclusions for the success or failure of the trial.

Bayesian sequential stopping rules for the design and conduct of clinical trials are outlined and developed in the later parts of the chapter, then the software developed at MDACC for the design of such trials is described. The focus will be on Bayesian stopping rules for safety and efficacy in Phase I, II, and III trials.

Lastly, several examples are presented. The first example is a Phase I trial in renal cell carcinoma that illustrates a Bayesian dose finding based on logistic regression, while the second is a hypothetical Phase II study developed by the author, but based on an actual study for inter-observer agreement in lung cancer. The third illustrates a statistical stopping rule for a Phase II trial in melanoma. For the three examples, the role of diagnostic imaging is emphasized.

8.2 Clinical Trials

8.2.1 Introduction

Thall,[1] who emphasizes the role that ethics and science play in the design and analysis of clinical trials, best explained the Bayesian methods in these trials. He stresses the complexity of such studies because they involve decisions for selecting therapies, the choice of dose levels of a particular regimen, and, above all, the concern for the patient's safety. Primarily for the concern for patient safety, clinical trials should be conducted in a sequential fashion, which calls for interim monitoring of patient outcomes.

This section will review the three phases of a clinical trial and focus on the role of diagnostic imaging in such studies. Later, Bayesian sequential stopping rules for interim analysis of clinical trials will be explained in more detail.

8.2.2 Phase I Designs

Phase I trials evaluate how a treatment is to be administered and how that treatment affects the human body. First, consider a Phase I study that evaluates safety among a set of doses of a new treatment. The study will be designed to determine the maximum tolerable dose (MTD), which is the dose whereby, at higher doses, the safety of the patient would be compromised. One is assuming that as the dose level increases, the probability of toxicity increases and also the probability of efficacy. The main endpoint in a Phase I study is various measures of toxicity experienced by the patient as a result of the treatment, while the secondary endpoint is various measures of efficacy. To define the toxicity endpoint, the investigator characterizes the dose limiting toxicity (DLT), which is a set of toxicities that are severe enough to prevent giving more of the treatment at higher doses. The investigator bases the DLT on knowledge of the disease, treatment, and the patients who are eligible for the trial. Investigators are guided by the National Cancer Institute (NCI) list of common toxicities or in some other manner that is appropriate for the particular study.

Prior to implementing a Phase I trial, the investigator must have decided upon the treatment route of administration and schedule. Also required for estimating the MTD are the patient population (defined via the eligibility and ineligibility criteria), a starting dose and a set of dose levels to test, the DLT, and the dose escalation. The dose escalation includes decisions of selecting the MTD among a set of doses. The chosen starting dose is based on other similar Phase I studies and/or information from animal experiments. Once the investigator has chosen the dose levels to be tested, the dose escalation can be described.

There are many dose-escalations rules, including the commonly used 3 + 3 design and the continual reassessment method (CRM). Since the early days of the NCI, investigators have used traditional escalating rules, such as the

3 + 3 design, for determining the MTD in oncology trials, while the CRM (see Crowley[2]) is a newer development that is becoming more popular. The 3 + 3 design is based on cohorts of size 3 or 6, and there are several versions.

What is the role of diagnostic imaging in Phase I clinical trials? The assessment of safety can include imaging of damage due to treatment and can also be an integral part of the assessment of efficacy. If a solid tumor is involved, imaging will measure the growth of that tumor during the course of the trial and this information will then be used in planning the Phase II trial and can serve as a source of prior information for a Bayesian sequential design. Since therapeutic trials most often use patients with advanced disease, there are many tumors per patient that will be imaged for change from start of treatment.

8.2.3 Phase II Trials

Once a particular treatment or intervention has been studied with a Phase I trial and the MTD has been selected and one is satisfied that the treatment will be safe, studies of the treatment may progress to Phase II trials to determine if the treatment holds sufficient promise. Typically, the target population is patients with a specific disease, disease site, histology, or stage, or patients undergoing some surgical or other procedure. Often the treatment dose is the MTD determined from previous Phase I trials. Although limited dose finding is sometimes allowed to accommodate different patient populations, the primary endpoints are measures of efficacy, while safety would be secondary.

It is in the Phase II trials that diagnostic imaging plays a crucial role. Often the primary endpoint is the fraction of patients who experience a response to therapy, and often the response is based on the change in tumor size as measured from baseline to some future point at the end of the treatment cycle. The response categories can be classified as a complete response, a partial response, or no response depending on the percent relative change from baseline. The WHO (World Health Organization) and RECIST criteria, as described by Padhani and Ollivier,[3] define the actual response categories that must be carefully specified in the protocol. It is important to understand the uncertainty introduced into such trials by the disagreement between the radiologists, who are responsible for assigning the response to therapy to each patient. This uncertainty is often unknown and unaccounted for by others, including statisticians, who are designing and analyzing trial information.

The efficacy information from a Phase I trial also is important and largely determines the type of Phase II trial to be designed. If little is known about the efficacy, a Phase IIa trial can be performed with the goal of determining a certain minimum efficacy. On the other hand, if the efficacy information from Phase I trials indicates that the intervention does indeed have some benefit, a Phase IIb trial may be implemented to determine if the treatment has sufficient benefit compared to some standard treatment, either historical (from past patient data) or from ongoing trials.

Reviewed below is how prior information from the relevant Phase I trials will be employed in the design of Bayesian sequential stopping rules and sample size information of the planning of the Phase II trial.

Designs for Phase IIa trials include Gehan's two-stage and Simon's[4] two-stage. Also relevant are multistage designs that are explained in Crowley.[2] Simon's two-stage is discussed here because it is the most popular for a Phase IIa trial; however, Bayesian alternatives are becoming more widely used because they are more flexible and can easily incorporate information from prior related Phase I and II trials.

Phase II designs are based on statistical testing principals. Suppose p is the probability of a treatment response, then one tests the null hypothesis vs. the alternative hypothesis:

$$H: p < p_0 \text{ (e.g., = .05)} \quad \text{vs.} \quad A: p \geq p_1 \text{(e.g., = .25)}.$$

The null hypothesis states that the proportion of responses is less than or equal to some specified proportion p_0 that would not exhibit sufficient interest for further development. The alternative hypothesis states that the proportion of responses is greater than or equal to a proportion p_1 that the investigator considers clinically meaningful. If the alternative hypothesis is true, then further testing could be deemed reasonable. Of course, this decision is based on other considerations as well, such as any new information on safety.

The values for p_0 and p_1 are specified in advance and depend on the results of previous trials. Typical values of p_0 are from .1 to .4, and typical values for p_1 are from p_0 + .15 to p_0 + .2. To use a Simon two-stage design, investigators must also specify the probability of a Type I error α, the probability of rejecting the null hypothesis when it is true (declaring that the new treatment has an effect above p_0 when it actually does not), and β, the probability of accepting the null hypothesis when it is false (declaring that the new treatment has no effect above p_0 when it actually does). Note that $(1 - \beta)$ is the power of the test.

Given these values, the Simon method will give the maximum sample size n, the stage 1 sample size n_1, and the rejection rule at each stage. DeVita et al.[5] provide tables for Simon's two-stage design. For example, when alpha = .05, beta = .20, p_0 = .05, and p_1= .25, then $n_1 = 9$, $n = 17$, and the trial would be stopped early if there were 0 out of 9 responses. If there were 1 or more responses with 9 patients, the trial is continued, and if there are 2 or fewer responses among 17 patients, the null hypothesis is accepted, that is, the intervention or treatment would not be of sufficient interest for further testing. With this design, the trial is stopped early for lack of efficacy. The Simon design can be used to justify the sample size and for stopping early. Stopping early protects future patients from receiving inefficacious treatments.

There are some Bayesian designs that allow more flexibility. For example, suppose the maximum sample size of N patients are accrued in k cohorts of size n and that, after observing the response of patients at the end of each cohort, the investigator computes the probability that the observed proportion of responses p is greater than p_1. If this probability is small, say,

.10 or .20, the trial is stopped for lack of efficacy. This is very much like the Simon design; however, a decision on lack of efficacy can be made after each cohort of patients. See Thall et al.[6,7] for additional information on Phase II trials that use Bayesian stopping rules.

If the intervention under investigation has shown some activity, a Phase IIb trial can be used to determine the extent of efficacy. This type of trial is usually comparative since it has demonstrated prior efficacy; the study intervention will be compared to some historical control or to some standard current treatment via a randomized design. The advantage of using historical controls over concurrent controls is the smaller number of patients required, but the disadvantages of historical controls are that the patient populations may not be comparable to those used in the current clinical trial.

8.2.4 Phase III Trials

We are now at the point where an intervention (drug or procedure) has been studied in a series of Phase I and Phase II trials and has demonstrated sufficient promise to be compared to the standard clinical treatment in a large randomized study.

Phase III trials are confirmatory where the study procedure is to be compared to the standard therapy with the goal of providing evidence that the study drug will provide substantial improvement in survival time or in disease free survival or some other time-to-event endpoint, such as time to response or time to hospitalization, etc. They should be designed to have a sufficient sample size to detect clinically relevant differences and are usually done in a multicenter setting. Provisions are made for interim looks by an independent Data Safety Monitoring Board where the trial may be stopped early for reasons of safety and/or efficacy. The response to therapy may serve as a secondary endpoint in Phase III trails, thus, diagnostic imaging plays a crucial role in the conduct of all clinical trials.

8.3 Protocol

What is a protocol? It states in detail how the medical study is to be organized and executed. There are generally two types: those submitted by a pharmaceutical or medical device company and those that are initiated by a principal investigator (PI) at the institution. The protocol should include the following components:

1. An explanation of the scientific basis for the study.
2. A summary of the results of all previous related studies and experiments of the study intervention.
3. The patient eligibility and ineligibility criteria.

4. A list of the major and minor endpoints, including their definitions and how and when they will be measured.
5. The definitions of evaluable and intent-to-treat populations.
6. The estimated patient accrual rates by site.
7. A statistical section that outlines a detailed power analysis for sample size, a description of rules for stopping early, methods for randomizing patients, and the proposed statistical analysis.
8. Nonstatistical stopping rules for safety considerations.

Additional documentation that must accompany the protocol is a list of all National Institutes of Health (NIH) toxicities and the patient-informed consent form. For protocols initiated by private companies, a biostatistician is assigned to review it, but for protocols initiated at MDACC, the study has one biostatistician assigned as a collaborator (the one who assisted the PI in the statistical design) and a different statistician who reviews it and presents it to the department for approval.

Every protocol at MDACC is reviewed in three stages: first by the Department of Biostatistics and Applied Mathematics, next by the Clinical Research Committee (CRC), and lastly by the Institutional Review Board (IRB). During the first review, a biostatistician presents the protocol in written and oral form to the department, and there is a set procedure for this presentation. The presentation is concluded with a list of major and minor concerns regarding the revision of the protocol. Then, the department discusses the abovementioned recommended revisions and votes to approve a directive to be sent to the PI. If need be, the PI then revises the protocol accordingly, often with the help of the biostatistical collaborator and/or reviewer.

8.4 Guidelines for Tumor Response

The RECIST criteria provide the radiologist with guidelines for determining the change in tumor size in such a way that the response to therapy can be judged and the success or failure of the trial evaluated. The following outline will be useful for understanding the guidelines: eligibility, methods of measurement, baseline identification of target and nontarget lesions, response criteria, evaluation of best overall response, confirmation and duration of response, and reporting of results.

Only patients with measurable lesions are eligible, namely those that can be accurately measured with computed tomography (CT) or magnetic resonance imaging (MRI). Both targeted and nontarget lesions are to be identified. A maximum of 10 lesions representative of all involved organs are identified as target lesions, which must be accurately and repeatedly measured by the longest diameter of the lesion. The primary endpoint is the sum of the longest diameters (SL) of the target lesions. All other lesions are identified as nontarget lesions. The RECIST criteria must take into account many tumors per patient because the patients in these trials usually have advanced disease, which has metastasized.

Based on the SL of the target lesions, each patient is classified into the following categories:

- Complete response (CR) where all target lesions disappear.
- Partial response (PR) where there is at least a 30% decrease in the SL of all target lesions using the baseline SL as a reference.
- Progressive disease (PD) where there is at least a 20% increase in the SL, relative to the smallest value of SL recorded since the treatment started.
- Stable disease (SD) where there is neither sufficient shrinkage to qualify as PR or sufficient increase to quality as PD.

There is also an evaluation of the nontarget lesions where the patient is classified as: complete response, incomplete response/stable disease, and progressive disease. The patient is then given an overall best response, based on the response of the target and nontarget lesions, and, finally, the patient is put into one of four overall categories: CR, PR, SD, and PD. (See Therasse et al.[8] for more detailed information on the RECIST guidelines and Padhani and Ollivier[3] for implications of those guidelines for diagnostic radiologists.)

The guidelines are only that and do not include the procedures of just how they are to be implemented. For example, there is no mention of the number of readers to be included or a procedure for the resolution of disagreement between radiologists in their determination of the patient's response to therapy. All of these elements create an element of uncertainty, which is unknown by others involved in the design and conduct of a clinical trail. This creates uncertainty in the classification of a patient's response to therapy and, consequently, is not accounted for by the statisticians in their design and analysis of Phase II clinical trials.

The study by Thiesse et al.[9] gives one some idea of the uncertainty in the process of assigning a patient's response to treatment. The study evaluated the impact of a review committee on the overall response status of a patient for a large multicenter trial with 489 patients for renal cancer given cytokine therapy (see Negrier et al.[10]). There were five response categories: CR, PR, MR, SD, and PD where MR stands for marginal response. The review committee completed a blinded peer review of all responders and all litigious cases. The results (Table 8.1) for 126 reviewed files are given in Thiesse et al.

Using the generalization of the G-coefficient (Chapter 7) Equation(7.3), its posterior distribution is easily found with Minitab® and provides a posterior mean of .019, a median of .018, and a standard deviation of .089. This implies that the agreement between the review committee and the original readers was very poor. Indeed, the Thiesse study itself gives .32 as the Kappa coefficient, which also confirms poor agreement. This indeed shows that

TABLE 8.1

Agreement between the Review Committee and the Original Report

	Response by Review Committee					
	CR	PR	MR	SD	PD	Total
Original Report						
CR	14	2	1	0	2	19
PR	4	38	4	6	10	62
MR	0	7	9	3	5	20
SD	0	0	1	4	15	20
PD	0	1	0	3	1	5
Total	18	48	11	16	33	126

disagreement among radiologists is quite common in the conduct of a clinical trial and, in particular, in the assignment of a patient's response to therapy.

Many studies have demonstrated such lack of agreement between radiologists. For example, a recent investigation of Erasmus et al.[11] shows the lack of consistency in measuring tumor size and poor intra- and inter-observer agreement. In fact, for some lesions, there was as much as a 50% difference in measuring the lesion size for two looks at the same image by the same reader.

8.5 Bayesian Sequential Stopping Rules

Due to the complexity of clinical trials and the incorporation of prior information from other previous studies, the Bayesian approach to interim analysis is quite appropriate. What is to be presented here is for Phase II trials where response to therapy is the primary endpoint, while toxicity is a secondary endpoint. Prior information on response and toxicity will be taken from previous Phase I and II trials that are relevant to the "new" therapy. The response to therapy is the main endpoint generated by radiologists using the RECIST criteria. The software to implement the design of the Bayesian stopping rule will be discussed and demonstrated in the next section.

Denote the following four probabilities of mutually exclusive and exhaustive events for a Phase II trial of an experimental therapy as: θ_1 = probability of response and toxicity, θ_2 = response and no toxicity, θ_3 = no response and toxicity, and θ_4 = no response and no toxicity. Suppose the corresponding probabilities of a previous standard relevant study are ϕ_1, ϕ_2, ϕ_3, and ϕ_4, respectively. Thus, the probability of a response with the experimental therapy is $\theta_r = \theta_1 + \theta_2$ and that for the standard is $\phi_r = \phi_1 + \phi_2$, the probability of toxicity with the experimental is $\theta_t = \theta_1 + \theta_3$,, while the probability for the standard is $\phi_t = \phi_1 + \phi_3$. It is known that $\theta = (\theta_1,\theta_2,\theta_3,\theta_4)$ and $\phi = (\phi_1,\phi_2,\phi_3,\phi_4)$ have Dirichlet distributions, thus, so do (θ_r, θ_t) and ϕ_r,ϕ_t.

Now suppose, based on historical information, that among n patients on the standard therapy, there are a responses, and among m patients, there are b toxicities, while for the "new" experimental therapy, *a priori*, there will be c responses and d toxicities.

Therefore, *apriori*, $\phi_r \sim beta(a, n-a)$ and $\phi_t \sim beta(b, m-b)$. Frequently, the prior information about experimental therapy is taken to be vague or non-informative, and one could let

$$\theta_r \sim beta(1,1) \quad \text{and} \quad \theta_t \sim beta(1,1).$$

The alternative hypothesis is

$$A\text{: } \theta_r < \phi_r \quad \text{or} \quad \theta_t > \phi_t \quad \text{vs.} \quad \text{the null } H\text{: } \theta_r \geq \phi_r \quad \text{and} \quad \theta_t \leq \phi_t.$$

The rule to stop the trial after observing the number of responses and toxicities is when

$$\Pr[\theta_r < \phi_r / data] > \eta \quad \text{or} \quad \Pr[\theta_t > \phi_t / data] > \varepsilon \tag{8.1}$$

where η and ε are usually selected "large," say, .90 or .95.

Thus, the trial is stopped if the posterior probability is high that the number of responses with the experimental therapy is less than that of the standard or if the posterior probability is large when the number of toxicities with the experimental therapy exceeds that of the standard. Since ϕ_r and ϕ_t are correlated, the events $\theta_r < \phi_r$ and $\theta_t > \phi_t$ are not independent!

Diagnostic imaging plays an important role for this type of trial. It is important to know how the trial parameters are based on prior information. Such information about efficacy, most likely, is the result of imaging the tumor size in Phase I trials. For the trial at hand, the number of responses and number of toxicities are based on imaging the size of the primary tumor and tumors at the sites of metastases. Note that θ_r (the probability of a response) is based on the RECIST criteria for categorizing patients into the various responses categories: CR, PR, SD, and PD. The protocol must specify the definition of response that is used in the Bayesian stopping rule. Usually, response means the event CR or PR, which, as has been explained above, depends on the change in tumor size from some reference time, defined in the protocol. The protocol will not mention the number of readers or how disagreements between readers are resolved. Of course, such information is not known to the statisticians, who assist in the analysis of the trial information.

The following example is taken from Cook.[12] Suppose a previous related trial had 200 patients, among which a = 60 responded and 140 did not. Among 160 of these patients, b = 40 experienced toxicities, but 120 did not experience any serious side effects. Let the prior distribution of $\phi_r \sim beta$ (60,140) and $\phi_t \sim beta(40,120)$, while the prior distributions for the corresponding parameters of the melanoma group for response and toxicity are assumed to be uniform.

TABLE 8.2

Stopping Rule for Response

Response	Boundary
0	6
1	12
2	17
3	22
4	27
5	30

The trial is stopped when the null hypothesis is rejected, namely when

$$\Pr[\theta_r < \phi_r/data] > .95$$

or (8.2)

$$\Pr[\theta_t > \phi_t/data] > .95.$$

The stopping rule for response is shown in Table 8.2

Thus, if there are no responses among the first six patients, the trial is stopped. One must know the response among at least six patients before the stopping rule for response takes effect. On the other hand, the stopping rule for toxicity is listed in Table 8.3. If the first three patients experience toxicity, the trial is stopped. What are the frequency properties of this test? Suppose the null hypothesis is "true" and that, hypothetically, $\theta_r = .4$, $\theta_r = .2$, $\phi_r = .3$, and $\phi_t = .25$, then using the above stopping rule, the probability of stopping the trial with various sample sizes is given in Table 8.4.

The probability of stopping is equivalent to the probability of a type I error. With only 3 patients, the probability is .008 of stopping the trial and, as the sample size increases, the probability of stopping slowly increases to 28 patients, then the probability has to increase to 1 at the maximum sample size of 30. Also for this scenario, the average number of patients is 26.7, experiencing an average of 5.34 toxicities and an average of 1.68 responses. The average number of patients treated is relatively large because this scenario occurs when the null hypothesis is true.

Now, suppose the alternative hypothesis is "true" with $\theta_r = .2, \theta_t = .35, \phi_r = .3$, and $\phi_t = .25$, then the probability of stopping is equivalent to the "power" of the test and is given in Table 8.5.

With this particular scenario of the alternative hypothesis, the probability of stopping or "power" gradually increases from .0429 with 3 patients to 1 with 30. The average number of responses is 2.8 with an average of 4.92 toxicities among an average of 14 treated patients. The probability of stopping or power is approximately .8 with 29 patients.

TABLE 8.3

Stopping Rule for Toxicity

Toxicity	Boundary
3	3
3	4
4	6
5	8
6	10
6	11
7	13
7	14
8	16
8	17
9	19
10	21
10	22
11	24
11	25
12	27
12	28
13	30

TABLE 8.4

Probability of Stopping: A Null Scenario $\theta_r = .4$, $\theta_t = .2$, $\phi_r = .3$, and $\phi_t = .25$

n	Probability of Stopping
3	.0080
4	.0272
5	.1037
6	.1095
8	.1120
9	.1128
11	.1198
12	.1268
13	.1277
14	.1298
16	.1305
17	.1355
19	.1361
20	.1375
22	.1395
23	.1406
25	.1409
26	.1430
28	.1433
29	.439
30	1.000

TABLE 8.5

Probability of Stopping: An Alternative Scenario $\theta_r = .2$, $\theta_t = .35$, $\phi_r = .3$, and $\phi_t = .25$

n	Probability of Stopping
3	.0429
4	.1265
5	.4235
6	.4517
8	.4680
9	.4980
11	.5132
12	.5798
13	.5881
14	.6044
16	.6125
17	.6713
19	.6780
20	.6902
22	.7261
23	.7361
25	.7409
26	.7763
28	.7802
29	.7874
30	1.000

Thus, for any scenario of the probabilities for response and toxicity of the experimental and standard therapies, the probability of stopping the trial can be computed. This allows one to estimate the sampling properties of the Bayesian test for stopping the trial.

8.6 Software for Clinical Trials

The Department of Biostatistics and Applied Mathematics at MDACC is developing many programs for the analysis and design of clinical and scientific studies in medicine and biology. These can be accessed at *http://Biostatistics/mdanderson.org/SoftwareDownload/*.

This library contains dozens of programs and are easily accessible to the student. Only two of the most relevant for clinical trials will be described. The first is appropriate for Phase I dose-finding trials, while the second is used for Phase II trials, when the major endpoints are for response and toxicity. The latter program is called Multc Lean and the former CRM Simulator.

8.6.1 CRM Simulator for Phase I Trials

Phase I trials are the beginning for the study of a new agent or therapy, and the first concern is for safety of the patient. The study is designed to determine the MTD, which is the dose whereby, at higher doses, the safety of the patient would be compromised. We are assuming that, as the dose level increases, the probability of toxicity increases and the probability of efficacy also increases. The main endpoint in a Phase I study is various measures of toxicity experienced by the patient as a result of the treatment, while the secondary endpoint is various measures of efficacy. To define the toxicity endpoint, the investigator specifies the DLT, which is a set of toxicities that are severe enough to prevent giving more of the treatment at higher doses. The investigator bases the DLT on knowledge of the disease, treatment, and the patients who are eligible for the trial. Investigators are guided by the NCI's list of toxicities or in some other manner that is appropriate for the particular study.

Also required for estimating the MTD is the patient population defined via the eligibility and ineligibility criteria, a starting dose and a set of dose levels to test, the DLT, and the dose escalation. The dose escalation plan includes decisions on how to select the MTD among a set of doses. The chosen starting dose is based on other similar Phase I studies and/or information from animal experiments. Once the investigator has chosen the dose levels to be tested, the dose escalation can be described.

The CRM simulator uses only one endpoint, namely toxicity, and is easily executed. The student should refer to the *CRM Simulator Guide* and *Methods of Description*. Both technical reports can be accessed from the above Internet address.

8.6.2 Multc Lean for Phase II Trials

The example of a Phase II trial in Section 8.5 was implemented using Multc Lean. There are two major endpoints: one for the number of responses and one for the number of toxicities among the maximum number of patients to be accrued for the trial. The methods is best explained by the "Multc Lean Statistical Tutorial" by Cook,[12] which together with the program, can be downloaded from the above address. The user must supply the maximum number of patients to be accrued, and information about prior related studies. Prior therapy is referred to as the standard therapy, while the therapy to be tested is referred to as the experimental therapy. Prior information about the new treatment is usually given as noninformative or vague, while that for the standard is more informative and usually provided with the number of responses and the number of toxicities experienced by a given number of patients in earlier Phase I studies.

Multc Lean consists of four parts: model input, stopping criteria, scenario input, and scenario output. The model input statement specifies the prior information for the standard and experimental treatments. With regard to the stopping criteria, recall from Section 8.5 that

$$\Pr[\theta_r < \phi_r / data] > .95$$

or (8.3)

$$\Pr[\theta_t > \phi_t / data] > .95.$$

The first probability is for stopping the trial when the probability of a response for the experimental therapy is less than that for the standard therapy. If this probability exceeds 95%, the trial is stopped for lack of efficacy, relative to the standard treatment. On the other hand, the trial is stopped if the probability of toxicity with the experimental treatment exceeds that of the standard with a high probability, in this case .95. All this information is specified in the stopping criteria section of Multc Lean. As a result of this information, the program provides stopping boundaries for response (Table 8.2) and toxicity (Table 8.3).

To know the frequency properties of the Bayesian stopping rule, Multc Lean computes the probability of stopping the trial for all sample sizes, given a particular scenario of values for $\theta = (\theta_1, \theta_2, \theta_3, \theta_4)$ and $\phi = (\phi_1, \phi_2, \phi_3\ \phi_4)$, and, therefore, for (θ_r, θ_t) and (ϕ_r, ϕ_t). The stopping criteria (Equation (8.2)) are given in terms of the response and toxicity parameters for the experimental (θ_r, θ_t) and standard (ϕ_r, ϕ_t) therapies, which must be kept in mind when running a particular scenario. For example, $\theta_r = .4$, $\theta_t = .2$, $\phi_r = .3$, and $\phi_t = .25$ was used when assuming the null hypothesis was true, while $\theta_r = .2$, $\theta_t = .35$, $\phi_r = .3$, and $\phi_t = .25$ was employed for an alternative hypothesis scenario. The program computes the probability of stopping, the average number of patients treated, the number of responses to be expected, and the average number of toxicities to be experienced by this average number of patients. (See Table 8.4 and Table 8.5 for the outcome of the two scenarios for the null and alternative hypotheses of this Phase II study.)

8.7 Examples

8.7.1 Phase I Trial for Renal Cell Carcinoma

Thall and Lee[13] describe three designs for Phase I trials. The 3 + 3, CRM, and Bayesian Logistic Regression are compared with regard to the percentage of times the correct dose is selected, and they use prior information to design a Phase I trial for renal cell carcinoma (RCC). Patients were previously treated with interferon and are to be treated with a fixed dose of 5-Fluorouracil (5-FU) and six dose levels of gemcitabine (GEM). These designs were briefly mentioned in Section 8.2.2, but only the latter design will be described and illustrated with WinBUGS®.

The logistic model for this design is

$$Log[\theta_i/(1-\theta_i)] = \alpha + \beta x_i$$

where there are d dose levels $x_1 < x_2 < ... < x_d$, θ_i is the probability of a dose-limiting toxicity at dose x_i, and α and β are unknown parameters. Recall that the objective of a Phase I trial is to estimate the MTD and to do this the investigator must specify the number of dose levels d, the dose level x_i, and a target toxicity level T. The MTD is that dose where the probability of toxicity is as close as possible to T. That is, doses greater than the MTD have probabilities of toxicity that are as least as large as T, while for doses that are less than the MTD, the corresponding probabilities of a dose-limiting toxicity are less than or equal to T.

Also to be specified is a rule for stopping the trial early. This can be problematic and there is no unique way to do it. One can choose n patients and test all n to estimate the MTD, or one can have a rule that stops the trial early if a given number of patients have been treated at the next recommended dose. Usually patients enter the trial in cohorts of size 3 or 6 and, after each cohort is treated, the next recommended dose level is selected.

The logit model assumes that as the dose level increases, so does the probability of a toxicity. However, it is usually true that as the dose level increases so does the probability of a favorable response, which creates somewhat of a dilemma, in that the two events, "toxicity" and "response," are competing with one another.

With the Bayesian approach, a prior probability for the parameters α and β must be specified, and this is usually done by selecting two probabilities of toxicity corresponding to two of the d dose levels, and "solving" the resulting two equations for α and β. This information is given by the study investigator and based on previous related human and animal studies. This way of estimating the MTD is taken from Thall and Lee (Table 1) and presented as Table 8.6. They assume the target toxicity level is $T = .25$ and do not use an early stopping rule, but use the information from all 36 patients.

The prior distribution for α and β are chosen so the probabilities of toxicity at doses 200 and 500 are .25 and .75, respectively, giving $\alpha = -1.1133$ and $\beta = .0031808$. This begins the process of selecting the MTD. With these initial values for the parameters as prior information, three patients enter the trial resulting in 0 toxicities, then the logistic model estimates the parameters and the six probabilities of toxicity corresponding to the six dose levels. The dose level 300 is the dose that has a probability of toxicity of .261, which is closest to the target toxicity level $T = .25$, thus 300 is selected as the next recommended dose. The process is repeated for the remaining 33 patients in cohorts of size 3. At the twelfth cohort, the next recommended dose level is 400, which is the estimated MTD. See the italicized numbers of Table 8.6.

It is important to remember that the primary aim of the Phase I trial is to provide information about the safety of the therapy, but an important secondary objective is to gather information on the efficacy of the treatment.

TABLE 8.6

Average Probability (%) of Toxicity by Dose of GEM (mg/m^2)

Cohort	Assigned Dose	Observed Number Toxicities	100	200	300	400	500	600
Prior			5.9	25	46.8	63.7	75	82.3
1	200	0	3.3	11.3	***26.1***	41.1	52.4	60.5
2	300	1	3.7	12.2	***29.1***	47.1	59.9	68.2
3	300	0	2.6	7.8	***19.2***	34.6	47.9	57.4
4	300	0	2.0	5.8	14.5	***27.7***	40.6	50.5
5	400	1	2.1	6.2	15.2	***29.4***	43.5	54.4
6	400	0	2.1	5.4	11.7	***21.7***	33.0	43.0
7	400	1	2.3	5.8	12.8	***23.9***	36.5	47.2
8	400	0	2.1	5.3	10.9	***19.9***	30.6	40.5
9	400	0	2.1	4.9	9.6	17.1	***26.4***	35.5
10	500	2	2.2	4.9	11.2	***22.4***	36.0	48.4
11	400	0	1.6	4.3	10.1	***20.1***	32.7	44.7
12	400	1	1.6	4.6	10.8	***21.3***	34.5	46.7

Source: Adapted from Thall, P.F. and Lee, S.J., *Int. J. Gynecol. Cancer*, 13, 251, 2003.

Both the estimated MTD and the information on efficacy will be used in any following Phase II trials. Diagnostic imaging will determine the response of the primary kidney tumor size and the response of the size of any metastatic lesions to treatment.

8.7.2 An Ideal Phase II Trial

As the first case of a Phase II trial that employs diagnostic imaging, Erasmus et al.[11] describe a hypothetical example based on real data. The study involves 5 readers, 40 lung cancer lesions, and 2 replications, that is, each reader views the same image twice. All readers read the 40 lesions and the major endpoint is the size of the lesion as determined by CT. The main focus of this study is to estimate the inter- and intra-observer error, and the main conclusion is that tumor size measurements are often inconsistent and can lead to incorrect interpretations of response to therapy based on the WHO and RECIST criteria.

Using the first replication of the five readers, the study results are used as baseline measurements for a hypothetical Phase II study. The first 10 lesions are used for patients with an intended complete response, and repeat measurements are assigned at random for times 1 and 2. The second set of 10 lesions is used for an intended partial response category of patients where the average lesion size decreased by 25% from time 0 to time 2. The basic descriptive statistics for the trial are given in Table 8.7.

A normal random number generator is used to generate hypothetical tumor size measurements by category of response and by the repeated measurement times 0, 1, and 2. Thus, for the complete response category of 10 patients, there was a 64% decrease in the average lesion size, relative to baseline. On the other hand, for the progressive disease category, the average lesion size increases from 3.95 centimeters to 4.94, an increase of 25.06%.

TABLE 8.7

Tumor Size Mean (sd) by Time and Response Category: Averaged over 10 Lesions

	Response			
	CR	**PR**	**SD**	**PD**
Time				
0	3.77 (1.57)	4.79 (.958)	4.20 (1.69)	3.95 (1.70)
1	2.16 (1.51)	4.26 (1.11)	4.14 (1.93)	4.34 (1.81)
2	1.37 (1.31)	3.81 (.947)	4.19 (1.68)	4.94 (1.70)
% Increase from baseline	–63.66	–20.45	.0023	25.06

There were five readers in this study and the mean (sd) readings for the three times are given in Table 8.8.

Each reader has 10 lesions for each of the 4 response categories. Assuming no disagreement between readers, how should their readings be used to assign lesions to response categories, CR, PR, SD, and PD? Suppose the lesions are assigned to two categories: response (including complete and partial response) if the percent decrease in lesion size is less than 30%; otherwise a lesion is assigned to the no response category.

Differences between readers will be tested with a logistic regression using the occurrence of response or no response as the dependent variable and using two factors for the independent variables: the patient label (1,2…,40) and the reader number (1,2,3,4). The logistic regression was performed using the WinBUGS statements below.

```
model
{
for(i in 1 : N ) {
y[i] ~ dbern(p[i])
logit(p[i]) <- beta[1] + beta[2]*n[i]+beta[3]*r[i]
}
phat <- mean(p[])
for (i in 1:3 ){
beta[i] ~ dnorm(0.0,0.0001)}
}
```

TABLE 8.8

Average (sd) Lesion Size for Five Readers by Time: Averaged over 40 Lesions

	Reader				
	1	**2**	**3**	**4**	**5**
Time					
0	3.92 (2.59)	3.70 (1.51)	4.42 (1.55)	4.36 (1.61)	4.14 (1.55)
1	3.48 (1.97)	3.09 (1.68)	3.83 (1.94)	3.92 (2.00)	3.56 (1.88)
2	3.24 (2.04)	3.02 (1.90)	3.72 (2.13)	3.64 (2.15)	3.37 (2.02)

TABLE 8.9

Posterior Distribution of Tumor Response

Parameter	Mean	SD	Median	95% Credible Interval
beta[1]	6.240	1.268	6.174	3.968, 8.906
beta[2]	–.459	.076	–.453	–.626, –.325
beta[3]	–.045	.214	–.045	–.471, .372
Phat: Overall response	.320	.016	.320	.287, .352

The list statement for the data includes the column *y*[] for the 200 occurrences of the overall response, while the *n*[] column contains the lesion id (1,2,…,40). The 200 by 1 reader id column is the coefficient of beta[3] in the logistic regression model. Zeros are given as the initial values of the three beta coefficients in the list statement for initial values of the program. The posterior analysis is given in Table 8.9. The lesion factor is included because the readers were paired with lesions, thus the effect for readers, given by beta[3], is adjusted for the lesion effect.

The lesion effect beta[2] is significant. Its 95% credible interval excludes zero; however, the interval for the reader effect does include zero, implying that reader differences have a minimal effect in estimating the tumor response phat. The posterior mean of the overall response is .32 with a standard deviation of .016 and a 95% credible interval of (.287, .352). Thus, the estimate of the overall response to therapy is 32%.

Of course, for the hypothetical outcomes of lesion size, the author designed the study so that there was good agreement between the readers.

8.7.3 Phase II Trial for Advanced Melanoma

Melanoma is a cancer of the skin and about 55,000 new cases are diagnosed annually culminating in approximately 8000 deaths. If not successfully treated in the early stage, it metastasizes to the brain, lungs, and liver, and, in this advanced stage, there are few promising therapies. The protocol to be explained is for Stage IV melanoma with a therapy that has shown some promise in other forms of cancer.

The therapy to be tested is an agent that is designed to be antiangiogenic (i.e., designed to destroy the blood supply to the tumor) and there have been several Phase I and Phase II trials that utilize this agent. In an early European Phase I trial with 37 patients with solid tumors, no serious toxicities were reported. In a Phase II study with 35 patients, this agent, in combination with another, produced no toxicities. In a NCI study with six patients, there were no objective responses, but three patients experienced stable disease. In an ongoing Phase II trial, there have been some minor toxicities and reports of one confirmed CR. Thus, prior information leads us to use the following: With 72 patients, there hasn't been any

TABLE 8.10

Overall Response to Therapy

Target Lesions	Nontarget Lesions	New Lesions	Overall Response
CR	CR	No	CR
CR	SD/incomplete response	No	PR
PR	Non-PD	No	PR
SD	Non-PD	No	SD
PD	Any	Yes or No	PD
Any	PD	Yes or No	PD
Any	Any	Yes	PD

reported serious toxicities and, at the same time, little evidence of a favorable response to therapy.

Patients to be entered into this study must have a confirmed stage IV disease, must have measurable disease with at least one lesion that can be accurately measured over the course of the study, be at least 18 years of age, and have a performance status that shows they are well enough to complete the therapy. This is a randomized study, with patients randomly assigned to two dose levels of chemotherapy where the endpoint is response to therapy.

In order to assign patients to a response category, the RECIST criteria (see Section 8.4) will be followed. A patient's overall response is based on dynamic CT scans of the target lesions. The final category is based on the imaging results for the target lesions, the status of the nontarget lesions, and the appearance of new lesions (Table 8.10).

In addition, the classification of response to the target lesions is based on the change (see Section 8.4) in lesion size for the target lesions, relative to some reference time, either at baseline or at some earlier time when the size of the lesion was minimum. One cycle of therapy is 4 weeks and the protocol must designate the times during this period when CT imaging of the target lesions will take place. Several treatment cycles of therapy must be experienced by patients in order for them to be assigned to an overall response category and for the category to be confirmed.

A statistics section of the protocol contains the power analysis, a justification for the sample size, and a description of the statistical analysis for the study results. It was decided that 57 patients could be accrued at the rate of 3 to 4 per month for this single center trial. A Bayesian stopping rule must be given that utilizes the information from prior Phase I and Phase II studies. We have seen that, with a total of 72 patients, no toxicities were reported and there was very little evidence of response to therapy (there were 3 of 6 who experienced SD in a European trial). Thus, there is good evidence of no toxicity, but very little evidence of response to therapy. Also, there is very little evidence for treatment response because these trials were designed primarily to evaluate safety, not efficacy, thus the prior information for response is designated as vague or uninformative.

TABLE 8.11

Prior Beta Distributions for the Standard and Experimental Therapies

Category	Therapy	Beta Parameters
Response	Standard	(1,1)
Response	Experimental	(1,1)
Toxicity	Standard	(1,71)
Toxicity	Experimental	(.0278, 1.9722)

Multc Lean is used to design the stopping rule for this trial. Table 8.11 shows that prior distribution is for the probabilities of response and toxicity of the standard and the melanoma trial.

Thus, one is quite confident that there was very little toxicity among the 72 patients of previous trials. A uniform prior is given to the probabilities of a response for the standard and experimental therapies. Using Multc Lean, the stopping rule is

$$\Pr[\theta_r < \phi_r / data] > .85$$

or (8.4)

$$\Pr[\theta_t > \phi_t / data] > .85$$

and the stopping boundaries for response are shown in Table 8.12.

The trial is stopped if there are 3 or less responses among the first 25 patients. On the other hand, Table 8.13 shows the stopping boundaries for toxicity and the trial is stopped early if the first patient experiences toxicity.

What are the sampling properties of this stopping rule? The third section of Multc Lean provides a way to estimate the probability of stopping for

TABLE 8.12

Stopping Boundaries for Response

Responses	Boundary
0	5
1	12
2	19
3	25
4	32
5	39
6	45
7	52
8	57

TABLE 8.13

Stopping Boundaries for Toxicity

Toxicity	Boundary
1	1–12
2	14–45
3	47–57

various scenarios involving the probabilities of response and toxicity of the experimental therapy relative to the corresponding probabilities of $\phi_r = .5$ [beta(1,1)] and $\phi_t = .0139$ [beta (1,71)] for the standard therapy. The five scenarios in Table 8.14 were assumed for the experimental therapy.

For each scenario, the probability of stopping for a given number of patients (Table 8.15) can be computed with Multc Lean. (See scenario input and output sections of the program.)

In addition, Multc Lean gives the average number of patients, the average number of responses, and the average number of toxicities for each scenario (Table 8.16).

TABLE 8.14

Scenarios of the Melanoma Study

Probability of Response θ_r	Probability of Toxicity θ_t	Scenario
.5	.5	1
.01	.01	2
.2	.2	3
.21	.02	4
.60	.011	5

TABLE 8.15

Probability of Stopping Early for Melanoma Trial

	Scenario				
n	1	2	3	4	5
1	.5000	.10000	.0200	.0200	.0110
5	.9697	.8532	.9548	.3848	.0639
10	.9999	.9133	.9592	.4439	.1143
20	1	.9867	.9994	.5654	.1366
40	1	.9994	1	.6442	.1666
56	1	.9998	1	.6707	.1795
57	1	1	1	1	1

TABLE 8.16

Average Number of Patients, Responses, and Toxicities

Scenario	Average Number of Patients	Average Number of Responses	Average Number of Toxicities
1	1.99	.999	.999
2	5.17	.517	.517
3	5.13	.102	.1076
4	26.29	5.52	.525
5	49.18	29.51	.541

8.8 Exercises

8.1 Verify the posterior analysis for the G-coefficient of Table 8.1. What is the posterior distribution of the Kappa parameter? See formula (7.6) in Chapter 7.

8.2 Using Multc Lean, verify the results of the Phase II trial of Section 8.5. See Table 8.2 to Table 8.5.

8.3 Verify Table 8.6 with a logistic regression written in WinBUGS.

8.4 Suppose a lesion is classified overall as a response if the percentage decrease in tumor size, relative to baseline, is less than 20%. Perform a logistic regression similar to that given in Table 8.9 and test for differences in readers.

8.5 Refer to Table 8.7 and generate lesion sizes, but where there are significant reader differences. How should the overall response be estimated in a Bayesian fashion?

8.6 Using Multc Lean, verify the results of the melanoma trial in Table 8.12 and Table 8.13.

8.7 Refer to Table 8.15 and explain the difference in the probability of stopping between scenarios 1 and 5.

8.8 By choosing different beta prior distributions for the parameters of the standard and melanoma therapies and using Multc Lean, describe the effect of the prior distribution on the probability of stopping the trial.

8.9 Refer to Table 8.16 and explain why the average number of patients for scenario 5 is much greater than that for scenario 1? What is the effect of the stopping probabilities on the average number of patients?

8.10 Refer to formula (8.3) where the probability of stopping for response and toxicity are both .85. Change these to .80 and .80, respectively, and determine the effect on the average number of patients, responses, and toxicities.

References

1. Thall, P.F., Bayesian methods in early phase oncology trials. *Proc. Sec. Bayesian Stat. Science*, 2000, The American Statistical Association.
2. Crowley, J., *Handbook of Statistics in Clinical Oncology*, Marcel Dekker, 2001, New York.
3. Padhani, A.R. and Ollivier, L., The RECIST criteria: implications for diagnostic radiologists, *Br. J. Radiol.*, 74, 983, 2001.
4. Simon, R., Optimal two-stage designs for Phase II clinical trials, *Control. Clin. Trials*, 1985, 10, 1, 1985.
5. DeVita, V.T., Hellman, S., and Rosenberg, S.A., *Cancer, Principles and Practice of Oncology*, 5th ed., Lippincott & Raven, 1997, New York.
6. Thall, P.F., Simon, R., and Estey, E.H., Bayesian sequential monitoring designs for single arm clinical trials with multiple outcomes, *Stat. Med.*, 14, 357, 1995.
7. Thall, P.F., Simon, R.M., and Estey, E.H., New statistical strategy for monitoring safety and efficacy in single arm clinical trials, *J. Clin. Oncol.*, 14, 296, 1996.
8. Therasse, P., Arbuck, S.G., Eisenhauer, E.A., et. al., New Guidelines to evaluate the response to treatment in solid tumors, *J. Nat. Cancer Inst.*, 92, 205,2000.
9. Thiese, P., Ollivier, L., DiStefano-Louieheau, D., Negrier, S., Savary, J., Pignard, K., Lesset, C., Escudier, B. Response rate accuracy in oncology trials: reasons for interobserver variability, *J. Clin. Oncol.*, 15, 3507, 1997.
10. Negrier, S., Escudier, B., Lasset, C., et al., The FNLCC CRECY trial: interleukin 2 (IL2) + interferon (IFN) in the optimal treatment to induce responses in metastatic renal cell carcinoma, *Proc. Am. Soc. Clin. Oncol.*, 15, 39, 1996.
11. Erasmus, J.J., Gladish, G.W., Broemeling, L.D., Sabaloff, B.S., Truong, M.T., Herbst, R.S., and Munden, R.F., Interobserver and intraobserver variability in measurement of non-small–cell carcinoma lung lesions: implications for assessment of tumor response, *J. Clin. Oncol.* 21, 2574, 2004.
12. Cook, J.D., *Multc Lean Statistical Tutorial*, Department of Biostatistics and Applied Mathematics , 2005, University of Texas MD Anderson Cancer Center.
13. Thall, P.F. and Lee, S.J., Practical model-based dose-finding in Phase I clinical trials: methods based on toxicity, *Int. J. Gynecol. Canc.*, 13, 251, 2003.

Chapter 9

Other Topics

9.1 Introduction

This final chapter of the book will present some additional advanced topics in statistical techniques that are employed for the analysis of data encountered in diagnostic medicine. For example, verification bias is an important topic that occurs when not all of the test results are subject to a gold standard. Screening for breast cancer is a good example of this. When the mammogram is positive, the patient is usually sent for biopsy, which serves as the gold standard. On the other hand, if the test result is negative, a biopsy is usually not performed. In such as situation, follow-up for those patients who test negative serves as the gold standard, however, this requires time and years can pass before the results are confirmed. This is a case of extreme verification bias and it is not possible to directly estimate the usual measures (true and false positive fractions) of test accuracy. Less extreme forms of verification bias occur when a certain percentage of negative test results are subject to the gold standard. For example, negative test results may be subject to the gold standard if there are other patient characteristics that put them at high risk.

Another form of bias occurs when the gold standard is not perfect, that is, when there is an imperfect reference standard. In many diagnostic imaging studies, the results of one imaging modality (e.g., CT) is "confirmed" by another modality (e.g., MRI or by PET/CT). In many such studies, the inaccuracy of the reference test is sometimes not taken into account in estimating test accuracy.

How is test accuracy measured in survival studies? Suppose there is a prognostic factor for survival, then how accurate is it in the prediction of survival? Of course, a Cox-regression analysis provides some information in this regard, but also one would like to have additional, more direct information about the correlation or association of the diagnostic test with survival. This will be explored using a Bayesian version based on an exponential survival distribution with censored observations that determines the association between median survival and the diagnostic test. An example taken from a melanoma study of Ekmekcioglu et al.[1] illustrates this idea.

Another variation of this problem is when the gold standard is not binary, but perhaps ordinal or continuous. Suppose one is measuring the size of a lesion via computed tomography (CT) with surgery as the gold standard. Then how is the area under the receiving operating characteristic (ROC) curves estimated? Obuchowski[2,3] proposes a method, which will be modified with a Bayesian approach.

Screening for disease was briefly mentioned in earlier chapters and will be developed in more depth here with reference to Bayesian approaches for estimating sensitivity and lead-time for periodic cancer screening.

Lastly, the Bayesian approach to decision theory in choosing an optimal therapy (taking the accuracy of imaging modality into account) is briefly described below, and the chapter concludes with a summary of the book and a section about future trends in diagnostic medicine.

9.2 Imperfect Diagnostic Test Procedures

We do not live in an ideal world and this applies to the world of diagnostic testing. For example, verification bias occurs when only a subset of the subjects undergoing testing are subject to the gold standard. Another form of bias is when the gold standard itself is not perfect. These situations are quite common and the student should be familiar with them. Bayesian methods that deal with these scenarios are introduced.

9.2.1 Extreme Verification Bias

A good example of testing, when only those that test positive are referred to the gold standard, is screening asymptomatic subjects for breast cancer with mammography. Those that have negative mammograms are usually not subject to a biopsy. Suppose that $Y = 0, 1$ indicates a negative and positive test result, respectively, and that $D = 0, 1$ indicates the absence and presence of disease, respectively, and that after screening 2000 women, there are 40 positive mammograms among those with disease (Table 9.1).

Only the 50 who test positive have a biopsy, while the 1950 who test negative do not. Therefore, the usual measures of test accuracy, true positive fraction

TABLE 9.1

Screening for Mammography

	Breast Cancer		
	$D = 0$	$D = 1$	Total
Test Result Y			
$Y = 0$	$?, \theta_{00}$	$?, \theta_{01}$	1950
$Y = 1$	$10, \theta_{10}$	$40, \theta_{11}$	50
			2000

TABLE 9.2

The Posterior Analysis of Detection Probability and False Referral Probability

Parameter	Mean	Median	SD	95% Credible Interval
DP	.020	.020	.003	.014, .026
FRP	.005	.005	.001	.002, .009

(TPF) and false positive fraction (FPF), are not directly estimable. However, the test results are still informative because the detection probability (DP)

$$DP = P[Y = 1, D = 1] \tag{9.1}$$

and the false referral probability (FRP)

$$\mathrm{FRP} = P[Y = 1, D = 0] \tag{9.2}$$

are estimable.

Assuming a uniform prior distribution for $\theta_{01}, \theta_{11}, (1 - \theta_{01} - \theta_{11})$, their joint posterior distribution is Dirichlet (11, 41, 1951), and the marginal distribution of $\theta_{00} + \theta_{01}$ is beta (1951, 51). The posterior analysis for the DP and FRP are given in Table 9.2.

The posterior analysis assumes that there are no observations in the (0,0) and (0,1) categories, and also assumes a uniform prior distribution for all three parameters. It is important to realize that there are no observations in these categories because the 1950 subjects that test negative do not undergo a biopsy. These patients will be followed and their disease status updated with time, but for the present analysis, there isn't any information on disease verification. Of course, there is very informative prior information available from other sources, which could be used in the analysis. Note that

$$DP = \rho \ \mathrm{TPF} \tag{9.3}$$

and

$$\mathrm{FRP} = (1 - \rho) \ \mathrm{FPF}, \tag{9.4}$$

and the usual estimators of TPF and FPF are easily obtained if one knows the disease prevalence = $P[D = 1]$. The prevalence cannot be estimated from the current study; however, such information is known with good credibility from other studies, and the posterior distribution of TPF and FPF easily computed.

Consider an example of diagnostic testing with a hypothetical screening study with 2000 subjects is experimental with both mammography and magnetic resonance imaging (*MRI*) testing for breast cancer, and that the

TABLE 9.3

Mammography and MRI for Breast Cancer

	MRI				
	D = 0	**D = 0**	**D = 1**	**D = 1**	**Totals Mammography**
Mammography					
	Y = 0	Y = 1	Y = 0	Y = 1	
Y = 0	?, θ_{00}	5, θ_{01}	?, ϕ_{00}	0,ϕ_{01}	1950
Y = 1	5, θ_{10}	5, θ_{11}	10,ϕ_{10}	30,ϕ_{11}	50
Totals MRI		10		30	2000

diagnostic score is subject to the gold standard when one or both tests are positive, with the results in Table 9.3.

This is a paired study with 2000 MRI and mammography images classified as positive or negative. When $Y=0$ for both images, the person is not referred to biopsy. An estimate of the DP for mammography is 40/2000 = .02 vs. 30/2000 = .015 for MRI, while the false referral rates are FRP = 10/2000 = .005 for both modalities.

Recall that for mammography, the diagnostic score is an ordinal confidence level with 5 values, where 1 indicates definitely not malignant and a 5 indicating definitely malignant. Values of 4 (probably malignant) and 5 are scored as positive for breast cancer. A similar scoring system is performed with MRI.

Assuming a uniform prior for η, the vector of all 7 parameters, gives a Dirichlet (6,6,6,1,11,31,1946) posterior distribution for

$$\tau = (\theta_{01}, \theta_{10}, \theta_{11}, \phi_{01}, \phi_{10}, \phi_{11}, \eta)$$

where

$$\eta = 1 - (\theta_{01} + \theta_{10} + \theta_{11} + \phi_{01} + \phi_{10} + \phi_{11}).$$

Note that the DP for mammography is

$$DP_{mamm} = \phi_{10} + \phi_{11}$$

and for the MRI is

$$DP_{mri} = \phi_{01} + \phi_{11},$$

while the FRPs are

$$FRP_{mamm} = \theta_{10} + \theta_{11}$$

and

$$FRP_{mri} = \theta_{01} + \theta_{11}.$$

TABLE 9.4

Posterior Distribution of τ

Parameter	Mean	Std
DP_{mamm}	.020	.003
DP_{mri}	.015	.002
FRP_{mamm}	.005	.001
FRP_{mri}	.005	.001
rTPF(mamm,mri)	1.321	.132
rFPF(mamm,mri)	1.045	.321

The TPF and FPF are not estimable individually, but the following ratios are:

$$\text{rTPF}(mamm,mri) = DP_{mamm}/DP_{mri}$$

and

$$\text{rFPF}(mamm,mri) = \text{FRP}_{mamm}/\text{FRP}_{mri}.$$

Thus, two modalities can be compared with the usual measures of test accuracy. Minitab® is used to determine the posterior distribution of τ with 1000 observations generated from the posterior distribution (Table 9.4).

The association between the detection probabilities of mammography and MRI are illustrated with a plot of the 1000 pairs generated from their joint posterior distribution given in Figure 9.1.

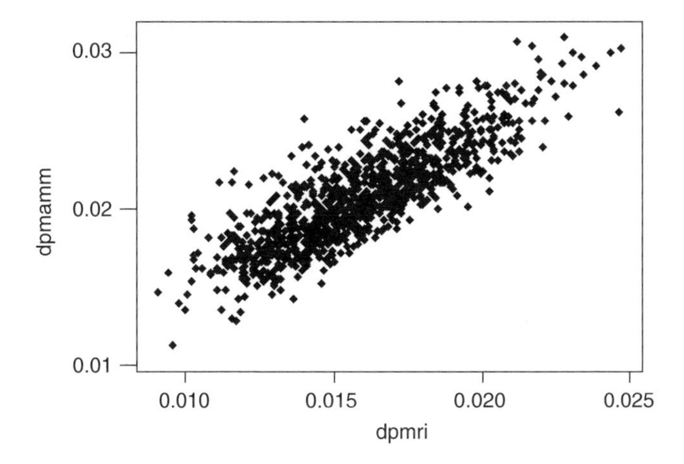

FIGURE 9.1
Detection probability of mammography vs. detection probability of MRI.

TABLE 9.5

National Lung Cancer Screening CT and X-Ray

Modality	$Y = 1, D = 0$	$Y = 1, D = 1$	$Y = 0$	Total
X-Ray	250	250	4500	5000
CT	100	400	4500	5000

Suppose a hypothetical national screening study for lung cancer is to be conducted with 10,000 present and former smokers aged 55 years and older. It will be a randomized study with 5000 allocated to X-ray imaging and CT. The anticipated results are shown in Table 9.5.

The anticipated detection probability for CT is 400/5000 = 8% compared to 5% with X-ray, and the percentage of positive results for both will be the same, namely 500/5000 = 10%. Note that 9000 participants who test negative will not have a biopsy for disease verification. The ongoing national lung cancer screening trial has 50,000 subjects (see Moore et al.[4])

9.2.2 Verification Bias

The examples above are an extreme form of verification bias in that all who test negative do not experience disease verification, but there are studies where among those that test negative, a certain fraction would be subject to the gold standard. This can occur with CT where the basic response is measured in Hounsfield units (a quantitative scale for describing radio density) and is used to measure heart disease. Values above a certain threshold indicate disease, while those below an absence. Suppose that an image is formally negative with the diagnostic score below the threshold, but there are other aspects of the image that might indicate a problem, whereas the subject is referred to the gold standard. An example of this is testing for coronary artery disease with a CT image that measures the amount of calcium in the coronary arteries.

There are other properties of the image that indicate the presence of the disease, even though the calcium level is below the threshold. Perhaps, the score is below the threshold, but on the high end, and to make sure, the radiologist refers the patient to an exercise stress test in order to verify the negative result.

Consider the example of verification bias in Table 9.6A, with 1250 patients over 60 years of age.

TABLE 9.6A

Fully Observed

Y	D = 0	D = 1	Total
$Y = 0$	900	100	1000
$Y = 1$	50	200	250
Total	950	300	1250

TABLE 9.6B

Verified Data

Y	D = 0	D = 1	Total
$Y = 0$	90, θ_{00}	10, θ_{01}	100
$Y = 1$	50,θ_{10}	200,θ_{11}	250
Total	140	210	350

The TPF = .667 and the FPF = .052, but suppose that 10% of those that test negative are subject to the gold standard, then there are 350 patients that have the disease status verified (Table 9.6B). When verification bias occurs, the results in Table 9.6A are not available.

The estimated TPF = .952 is larger than it should be, as is the FPF = .357, when compared to the .052 from the fully observed information.

Is it possible to determine reliable estimates of TPF and the FPF? It is possible under the MAR (missing at random) assumption. This states that the test negative patient is referred to the gold standard based only on the test results Y. The key word is "only" in that the decision to refer a test negative patient for disease verification cannot be based on considerations other than the test result, such as, for example, other symptoms of the patient or the fact that the patient might or might not belong to a high-risk group.

The MAR assumption is

$$P[D = 1/V = 1,Y] = P[D = 1/Y], \tag{9.5}$$

which implies the prevalence of disease in the population, from which the study group is selected, is the same as among those patients who are verified for disease. This is another way of saying that the decision to refer a subject for verification must depend only on the test result Y. It is easy to see why it would be difficult to verify the MAR assumption. It would be necessary to know the mind of the radiologists who are interpreting information from the images and others who are making the referral decision. Presumably, the radiologist is using all reliable information in the decision to refer a patient to the gold standard.

But, supposing MAR is true, how is it used to estimate the TPF and FPF from the selected data? The answer is Bayes theorem, namely

$$P[Y = 1/D = 1] = P[D = 1/Y = 1, \quad V = 1]P[Y = 1]/P[D = 1] \tag{9.6}$$

where $V = 1$ indicates the case is verified and

$$P[D = 1] = P[D = 1/Y = 1, \quad V = 1]P[Y = 1]+P[D = 1/Y = 0, \quad V = 1]P[Y = 0].$$

But, the MAR assumption implies $P[D = 1/Y = 1] = P[D = 1/V = 1,Y = 1]$, thus the information from the verified data in Table 9.6B can be used to

TABLE 9.7

Verified and Unverified Results

Test Result	$V = 1, D = 0$	$V = 0, D = 0$	$V = 1, D = 1$	$V = 0, D = 1$	Total
$Y = 0$	90, θ_{010}	810,θ_{000}	10,θ_{001}	90,θ_{001}	1000
$Y = 1$	200,θ_{110}		50,θ_{111}		250

estimate the positive predictive value $P[D = 1/Y = 1]$ and, hence, the TPF. For the example, the TPF is estimated as

$$\text{TPF} = .8(.25)/[.8(.25) + .10(.75)] = .727,$$

which is the approximate estimate from the fully observed in Table 9.6A.

In order to find the posterior distribution of the TPF, consider Table 9.7 where

$$\theta_{ijk} = P[Y = i, \quad D = j, V = k], \quad \text{and} \quad i, j, k = 0,1.$$

Let

$$\phi_{11} = P[D=1, \quad Y=1/V=1] = P[Y=1, \quad D=1, \quad V=1]/P[V=1] = \theta_{111}/(\theta_{111}+\theta_{110})$$

and

$$\phi_{01} = P[D = 1, Y = 0/V = 1] = \theta_{011}/(\theta_{010} + \theta_{011}),$$

then

$$\text{TPF} = \phi_{11}/(\phi_{11} + \phi_{01}). \tag{9.7}$$

Assuming a uniform prior density for the parameters, the posterior analysis is performed with Minitab using the information from Table 9.7. One thousand observations are generated from the joint posterior distribution of the parameters, with the results given in Table 9.8.

Begg and Greenes[5] derived asymptotic formulas for the confidence intervals of the TPF and FPF, but the Bayesian intervals are exact. Pepe[6] also provides several examples of using these formulas.

TABLE 9.8

Posterior Distribution of the TPF with Verification Bias

Parameter	Mean	Std	95% Credible Interval
TPF	.656	.068	.531, .790

TABLE 9.9

Imputed Data (Data of Table 9.6A)

Y	D = 0	D = 1	Total
$Y = 0$	900, γ_{00}	100 γ_{01}	1000
$Y = 1$	50, γ_{10}	200 γ_{11}	250
Total	950	300	1250

Of course, the test accuracy can also be computed from the data imputed from the verified data of Table 9.6b by multiplying the cell totals of the row with $Y = 0$ by the factor $1/P[V = 1] = 1/.10 = 10$. Consider the findings in Table 9.9 where

$$\gamma_{ij} = P[Y = i, D = j] \quad \text{and} \quad i, j = 0,1.$$

9.2.3 Estimating Test Accuracy with No Gold Standard

Joseph et al.[7] introduces a Bayesian approach to estimating disease prevalence, sensitivity, and specificity when there is no gold standard to verify the results of a diagnostic test. The analysis is illustrated with an example of two tests that diagnose *Strongyloides* infection in a group of Cambodian refugees arriving in Montreal, Quebec, over an 8-month period. The results are shown in Table 9.10.

Thus, serology and the stool examination both test positive for 38 subjects, with serology giving a prevalence 125/162 = 77% and 25% with the stool examination; a result not untypical of the two ways to diagnose the infection.

First, the serology test is considered, where Joseph et al. employ latent variables for the Bayesian approach. Suppose that when the disease is present, y_1 individuals out of 125 test positive and y_2 out of 37 test negative (Table 9.11) where $y_1 = 0,1,\ldots,125$, $y_2 = 0,1,\ldots,37$, and $\theta_{ij} = P(Y = i, D = j)$ where $i, j = 0,1$. The use of latent variables allows one to create hypothetical scenarios of disease detection when the disease is present.

TABLE 9.10

Testing for *Strongyloides Stercoralis* in 162 Refugees in Montreal

	Stool Exam		
	$Y = 1$	$Y = 0$	Total
Serology			
$Y = 1$	38	87	125
$Y = 0$	2	35	37
Total	40	122	162

TABLE 9.11

Latent Variables for Serology

Serology	$D = 1$	$D = 0$	Total
$Y = 1$	y_1, θ_{11}	$(125 - y_1), \theta_{10}$	125
$Y = 0$	y_2, θ_{01}	$(37 - y_2), \theta_{00}$	37
Total	$y_1 + y_2$	$162 - y_1 - y_2$	162

The Bayesian analysis consists of combining the likelihood function with the prior distribution for the unknown parameters p, s, and c for the prevalence, sensitivity, and specificity, respectively. The likelihood function is

$$L(\theta/data) = \theta_{11}{}^{y_1}\theta_{10}{}^{(125-y_1)}\theta_{01}{}^{y_2}\theta_{00}{}^{(37-y_2)}$$

where

$$\theta = (\theta_{11}, \theta_{10}, \theta_{01}, \theta_{00}).$$

Note that p is the prevalence and s the sensitivity, thus, the likelihood function is

$$L(p,s,c/data) = p^{y_1+y_2}(1-p)^{162-y_1-y_2} s^{y_1}(1-s)^{y_2} c^{37-y_2}(1-c)^{125-y_1} \tag{9.8}$$

where $0 \le p \le 1, 0 \le s \le 1$, and $0 \le c \le 1$. The specificity of the test is denoted by c.

Prior information about prevalence p and the sensitivity and specificity of serology is based on expert opinion of the McGill University Center of Tropical Diseases (Montreal, Canada) and summarized as follows:

$$p \sim \text{beta}(1,1),$$

$$s \sim \text{beta}(21.96,5.49),$$

and (9.9)

$$c \sim \text{beta}(4.1,1.76),$$

thus, the average sensitivity is expected to be 21.96/(21.96 + 5.49) = .80 and the expected specificity expected to be .70. Very little is known about the prevalence of the infection, therefore, a uniform prior is selected for p. Combining the likelihood function in Equation (9.8) with the prior information in Equation (9.9) via Bayes theorem gives the joint posterior distribution of p, s, and c.

The following statements allow one to perform the posterior analysis.

```
model;
# this analysis is based on Joseph et al. (1995)
{
y1~dbin(d,a)
# is the conditional distribution of y1 given y2, p, s,
and c
y2~dbin(e,b)
# is the conditional distribution of y2 given y1, p, s,
and c
p~dbeta(alp,bep)
# is the conditional distribution of p given y1, y2, s,
and c
s~dbeta(as,bs)
# is the conditional distribution of s, given y1, y2,
p, and c
c~dbeta(ac,bc)
# is the conditional distribution of c, given y1, y2,
p, and s
d<-p*s/(p*s+(1-p)*(1-c))
# d is the probability parameter of the distribution of
y1
e<-p*(1-s)/(p*(1-s)+(1-p)*c)
# e is the probability parameter of the distribution of
y2
alp<-y1 + y2 + alphp
# alp is the alpha parameter of the distribution of p
bep<-a + b - y1 - y2 + betp
# bep is the beta parameter of the distribution of p
as<-y1 + alphs
# as is the alpha parameter of the distribution of s
bs<-y2 + bets
# bs is the beta parameter of the distribution of s
ac<-b-y2+alphc
# ac is the alpha parameter of the distribution of c
bc<-a-y1+betc
# bc is the beta parameter of the distribution of c
}
```

```
list(a = 125, b = 37, alphp = 1,betp = 1,alphs = 21.96,
bets = 5.49, alphc = 4.1, betc = 1.76)
# gives the values for the parameters of the
distributions
list(y1 = 60, y2 = 8, p = .5, s = .5,c = .5)
# gives the starting values for the distributions
```

TABLE 9.12

Posterior Distribution of Test Accuracy of Serology

Parameter	Mean	Median	SD	95% Credible Interval
Sensitivity	.829	.829	.050	.733, .926
Specificity	.608	.621	.203	.230, .946
Prevalence	.796	.845	.181	.254, .990
*Y*1	108.2	117	23.04	34,125
*Y*2	21.62	22	9.068	4,37

The posterior distribution of p, s, and c is provided in Table 9.12.

The posterior analysis agrees very well with Joseph et al. The sensitivity is good, the specificity only fair, but the information about p is quite informative.

Figure 9.2 illustrates the posterior density of the sensitivity of the serology test for *Strongyloides.*

According to Table 9.12, the standard deviation of specificity is much larger than the standard deviation of the posterior distribution of sensitivity, thus, one is less confident about the estimated value .608 for specificity compared to .82 for sensitivity. Figure 9.2 and Figure 9.3 confirm this.

The Bayesian approach to test accuracy is easily extended to two diagnostic tests for infection. The results for both tests are given in Table 9.10. Table 9.13A and Table 9.13B display the results when the latent variables are included.

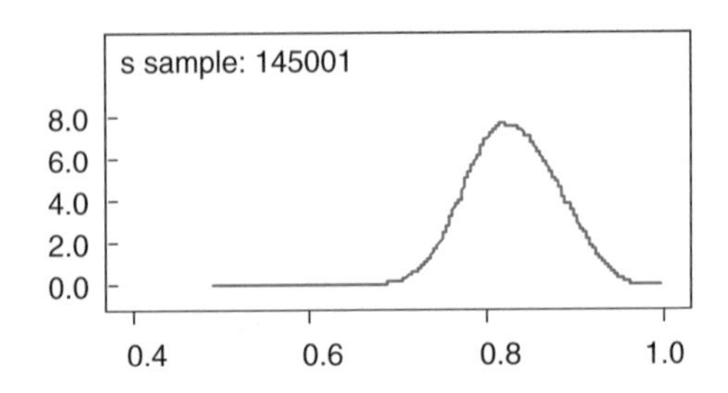

FIGURE 9.2
Posterior density of sensitivity of serology.

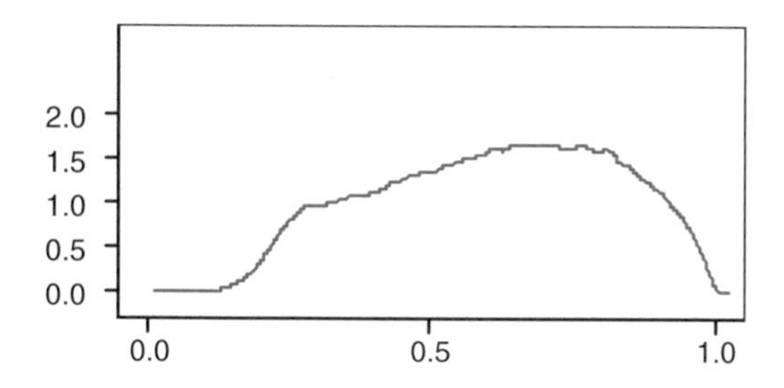

FIGURE 9.3
Posterior density of specificity of serology.

Assuming conditional independence between the two tests, it can be shown that the likelihood function is

$$L(p, c_1, c_2, s_1, s_2/data) = p^{y_1+y_2+y_3+y_4}\ s_1^{y_1+y_2}\ s_2^{y_1+y_3}\ (1-s_1)^{y_3+y_4}\ (1-s_2)^{y_2+y_4}$$

$$c_1^{37-y_3-y_4}\ c_2^{122-y_2-y_4}\ (1-c_1)^{125-y_1-y_2}\ (1-c_2)^{40-y_1-y_3} \tag{9.10}$$

where c_1 and c_2 are the specificities for stool and serology, respectively, and s_1 s_2 are the corresponding sensitivities, while p is the prevalence of *Strongloides.*

Note that the sensitivity, specificity, and prevalence are restricted to [0,1], and the ranges for the latent variables are $y_1 = 0, 1,\ldots, 38$; $y_2 = 0,1,\ldots,87$; $y_3 = 0,1,\ldots,2$; and $y_4 = 0,1,\ldots, 35$.

TABLE 9.13A
Stool and Serology: $D = 1$

	Stool Exam		
	$Y = 1$	$Y = 0$	Total
Serology			
$Y = 1$	y_1	y_2	$y_1 + y_2$
$Y = 0$	y_3	y_4	$y_3 + y_4$
Total	$y_1 + y_3$	$y_2 + y_4$	$y_1 + y_2 + y_3 + y_4$

TABLE 9.13B
Serology and Stool: $D = 0$

	Stool Exam		
	$Y = 1$	$Y = 0$	Total
Serology			
$Y = 1$	$38 - y_1$	$87 - y_2$	$125 - y_1 - y_2$
$Y = 0$	$2 - y_3$	$35 - y_4$	$37 - y_3 - y_4$
Total	$40 - y_1 - y_3$	$122 - y_2 - y_4$	$162 - y_1 - y_2 - y_3 - y_4$

9.3 Test Accuracy and Survival Analysis

Often a diagnostic test is also a prognostic factor for survival. For example, inducible nitric oxide synthase (iNOS) is used to diagnose metastasis of melanoma from the primary lesion to the lymph nodes, and from the lymph nodes to the other sites, such as the liver and lungs. Initially, Ekmekcioglu et al.[1] described the biological activity of iNOS and its prognostic value for overall survival of patients measured from their stage III diagnosis. Figure 9.4 shows the Kaplan–Meier plot comparing groups of patients, those who have an iNOS score of 0 vs. those with an iNOS score of 1.

A Bayesian analysis based on the exponential distribution gives a median survival for the iNOS = 0 group as 117 (26.2) months while, for the remaining patients, it is estimated as 30.49(4.39). The complete analysis is provided in Table 9.15.

Suppose T is the survival time with an exponential distribution with parameter λ and density

$$f(t) = \lambda \exp - \lambda t$$

where

$$t \geq 0. \tag{9.11}$$

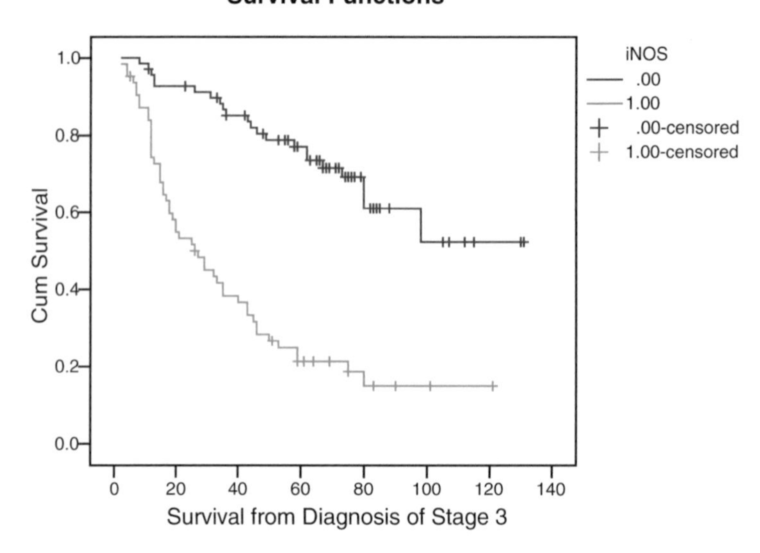

FIGURE 9.4
Kaplan–Meier plots for iNOS.

If there are r noncensored observations with survival times $t_1 \le t_2 \le \ldots t_r$ and $n - r$ censored observations at times $t_1^+ \le t_2^+ \le \ldots t_{n-r}^+$, then the likelihood function for λ is

$$L(\lambda/data) \propto \lambda^r \exp - \lambda\left(\sum_{i=1}^{i=r} t_i + \sum_{i=1}^{i=n-r} t_i^+\right). \tag{9.12}$$

Assuming a noninformative prior for λ, $f(\lambda) \propto 1/\lambda$,

$$\lambda / data \sim \text{gamma}, \left(r, \sum_{i=1}^{i=r} t_i + \sum_{i=1}^{i=n-r} t_i^+\right). \tag{9.13}$$

Since the mean survival time is $1/\lambda$ and the median survival time is $ln(1/2)/\lambda$, their posterior distributions are easily determined for those with iNOS = 0 and iNOS = 1.

From the Ekmekcioglu et al. study with 132 patients, the survival times and censored times for both populations are given in Table 9.14. Based on this table and the following program, the posterior analysis is given in Table 9.15.

TABLE 9.14

Survival Times for iNOS Groups

Censored	iNOS Score	r	$n - r$	$\sum_{i=1}^{i=r} t_i$	$\sum_{i=1}^{i=n-r} t_i^+$
no	0	22		981	
yes	0		47		3434
no	1	50		127	
yes	1		13		391

TABLE 9.15

Posterior Analysis for iNOS

Parameter	Mean	SD	Median	95% Credible Interval
Median 0	117	26.2	113.3	76.47, 179.0
Median 1	30.49	4.39	30.09	23.07, 40.28
Mean 0	168.8	37.8	163.5	110.3, 256.8
Mean 1	43.99	6.33	43.42	33.28, 58.12
Ratio Median	3.919	1.045	3.772	2.309, 6.385

```
model;
# exponential survival with censored obs
# based on Ekmekcioglu et al. (2006)
# m0 is mean survival for iNOS = 0
```

```
# m1 is mean survival for iNOS = 1
{  lambda0 ~ dgamma(a0, b0)
lambda1 ~ dgamma(a1, b1)
m0<-1/lambda0
m1<-1/lambda1
diffmean<- m0-m1
median0<-.6931/lambda0
median1<-.6931/lambda1
diffmedian<- median0-median1
ratiomedian<-median0/median
}
list(a0 = 22, b0 = 3542, a1 = 50, b1 = 2151)
list(lambda0 = 7, lambda1 = 7)
```

Of course, a Cox proportional hazard model gives a measure of association between iNOS and overall survival; however, the above posterior distribution for the ratio γ of the median survival times also provides an estimate. Indeed

$$\gamma = median0 / median1 \tag{9.14}$$

has a posterior mean of 3.919(1.045) with a 95% credible interval of (2.309, 6.385). Note that γ is positive and has a range of $(0, \infty)$ where values close to 1 indicate a weak association between survival and iNOS. On the other hand, values of γ less than 1 and large values greater than 1 indicate a stronger association between the two iNOS groups and the survival times.

This approach is quite different from Pencina and D'Agostino[8] who develop a ROC-type value that measures the concordance between a diagnostic score and the corresponding survival times.

9.4 ROC Curves with a Non-binary Gold Standard

There are many cases when the gold standard is not binary. For example, suppose one is using CT to estimate the size of lung lesions where surgery is the gold standard. This is a case where the gold standard is continuous. Obuchowski[2] gives an example of a continuous gold standard comparing the diagnostic accuracy of several tests that estimate blood iron concentrations. Serum ferritin is the gold standard used to verify the accuracies of two tests: percent transferrin saturation and total binding capacity. This example will be used to demonstrate the Bayesian approach.

The Bayesian approach is a modification of a nonparametric approach of Obuchowski, who defines the estimated ROC area for N patients as

$$\hat{\theta} = [1/N(N-1)]\sum_{i=1}^{i=N}\sum_{j=1}^{j=N}\varphi(x_{it}, x_{js}) \tag{9.15}$$

where x_{it} is the diagnostic score of the ith patient with a gold standard value of t. Also, the kernel $\varphi = 1$, if $t > s$ and $x_{it} > x_{js}$ or $s > t$ and $x_{js} > x_{it}$. In addition, $\varphi = .5$ if $t = s$ or $x_{it} = x_{js}$, and $\varphi = 0$ otherwise.

The interpretation of Equation (9.15) is familiar. It is the probability that a person with a higher gold standard outcome has a larger diagnostic score than a person with a lower gold standard score. For a given study, the value of $\hat{\theta}$ and its estimated standard deviation are known, and used to compute the parameters of the posterior distribution of the ROC area. Obuchowski provides an Internet address to download a Fortran program.

The variance of the estimator is

$$Var(\hat{\theta}) = [1/(N/2)(N/2-1]\sum_{i=1}^{i=N}[V(x_{it}) - \hat{\theta}]^2 \tag{9.16}$$

where

$$V(x_{it}) = [1/(N-1)]\sum_{j=1}^{j=N}\varphi(x_{it}, x_{js}),\ i \neq j \quad \text{and} \quad s = t. \tag{9.17}$$

The posterior distribution of the ROC area is assumed to be

$$\theta \sim \text{beta}(a,b) \tag{9.18}$$

where a and b parameters given by

$$a = vm$$

and

$$b = v(1-m),$$

with $m = \hat{\theta}$, and $v = 1/\hat{sd}(\hat{\theta})$.

The iron concentration study (with total binding capacity as the diagnostic test) of Obuchowski[2] is used to illustrate the Bayesian approach. Based on 55 female subjects, $\hat{\theta} = .829$ and $\hat{sd}(\hat{\theta}) = .025$, which gives $a = 33.12$ and $b = 6.88$. The simple program below provides the estimated area and its standard deviation as .829(.058), with a 95% credible interval (.699, .925). Note that a and b are the parameters of the posterior distribution, thus, prior information about the area can be easily expressed. In the example, a uniform prior was used for θ.

```
model;
{#Obuchowski
auc~dbeta(a,b)
# auc is area under the ROC curve
}
list(a = 33.12, b = 6.88)
# a and b are parameters of the posterior of auc
list(auc = .5)
# auc = .5 is starting value
```

9.5 Periodic Screening in Cancer

To introduce the Bayesian approach to estimating sensitivity for the screening of breast cancer with mammography, the recent results from Wu et al.[9] are reported. This is followed by a description of a similar study (Wu et al.[10]) for the estimation of the lead-time distribution for screening of the same disease. Both inferences are illustrated in the Health Insurance Plan of Greater New York (HIP) dataset.

9.5.1 Inference for Sensitivity and Transition Probability

In the first study, the goal is to estimate the age-dependent sensitivity and the transition probability (from the disease-free to the preclinical stage) in periodic screening for breast cancer. The fundamental model for screening consists of three stages, $S_0 \rightarrow S_p \rightarrow S_c$. Starting with the disease-free stage, passing to the preclinical, and finally entering the clinical stage of breast cancer where symptoms are displayed. Mammography is employed in the disease-free and preclinical stages and when the disease is detected in the preclinical phase, it allows for earlier treatment and longer survival for the subject. (See Berry et al.[11] for an account of the survival benefits from mammography screening.)

Based on studies of Zelen[12], Lee and Zelen[13], and Shen and Zelen[14], Wu et al.[9] developed a Bayesian approach to estimating the transition probability, from the disease-free to the preclinical stage, and the age-dependent sensitivity for periodic screening. Suppose a group of asymptomatic women are about to enter a screening program. Let $w(t)dt$ denote the transition probability from S_0 to S_p and let $q(.)$ denote the probability density of the sojourn time in the preclinical stage. Also let $\beta(t)$ be the sensitivity (the probability the mammogram is positive, conditional on being in the preclinical stage) of the test for an individual aged t, who is about to enter a screening program that is designed to have K-ordered examinations. The individual undergoes examinations at ages $t_0 < t_1 < ... < t_{K-1}$ where the ith screening interval is defined as the time between the ith and $(i + 1)$-st exam and define the ith generation as those who enter S_p at the ith screening exam. The $0th$ generation are those that enter the preclinical stage before the first examination, and $t_{-1} = 0$.

The HIP study recruited 62,000 women who were randomized into the study and control groups where the subjects in the former underwent four annual screening exams with mammography plus a clinical examination for breast cancer. For those in the control group, it was standard care. For the HIP data, there are 25 age groups corresponding to ages 40 through 64, thus, let $t_0 = 40, 41, ..., 64$, and suppose the exams are annual, that is, $t_{k-1} = t_0 + k - 1$. Suppose $n_{i,t0}, s_{i,t0}$, and $r_{i,t0}$ denote the total number of individuals in the group who entered the study at age t_0 and are undergoing the ith exam, the number of these who were detected with disease, and the number who were in the clinical stage within (t_{i-1}, t_i), respectively. The probability that a person in the S_p stage will be detected for disease at the initial exam is

$$D_{i,t_0} = \beta(t_0)\int_0^{t_0} w(x)Q(t_0 - x)dx \tag{9.19}$$

where $Q(z) = \int_z^\infty q(x)dx$ is the survivor function for the sojourn time in the preclinical stage.

In a similar fashion, consider a woman of the ith generation who was detected at the kth screening exam, which she did at age t_{k-1}, then either (a) she was undetected at the previous exams (k – i – 1) and had a sojourn time of at least $t_{k-1} - x$ where $x \in (t_{i-1}, t_i)$ is her age at entry into S_p or (b) she entered S_p in the (k – 1)-st screening interval (t_{k-2}, t_{k-1}).

Therefore,

$$D_{k,t_0} = \beta(t_{k-1})\left\{\sum_{i=0}^{i=k-2}[1-\beta(t_i)]\ldots[1-\beta(t_{k-2})]\int_{t_{i-1}}^{t_i} w(x)Q(t_{k-1}-x)dx + \int_{t_{k-2}}^{t_{k-1}} w(x)Q(t_{k-1}-x)dx\right\} \tag{9.20}$$

for $k = 2, \ldots, K$.

Suppose $I_{k,t0}(t)dt$ denotes the probability that a woman enters the clinical stage within $(t, t + dt)$ where $t \in (t_{k-1}, t_k)$. If the individual is in generation i, then $i < k$ and she must have gone undetected in her $(k - i)$ previous screenings and had a sojourn time of $(t - x)$, where x was her age of entry into S_p.

Another possibility is that she entered the preclinical stage after the k*th* exam and developed clinical disease at time t. This implies

$$I_{k,t_0}(t) = \sum_{i=0}^{i=k-1} [1-\beta(t_i)]\ldots[1-\beta(t_{k-1})] \int_{t_{i-1}}^{t_i} w(x)q(t-x)dx + \int_{t_{k-1}}^{t_k} w(x)q(t-x)dx \quad (9.21)$$

where $t \in (t_{k-1}, t_k)$.

Furthermore, the probability of being incident in (t_{k-1}, t_k) is

$$I_{k,t_0} = \int_{t_{k-1}}^{t_k} I_{k,t_0}(t)dt = \sum_{i=0}^{k-1} [1-\beta(t_i)]\ldots[1-\beta(t_{k-1}] \int_{t_{i-1}}^{t_i} w(x)[Q(t_{k-1}-x) - Q(t_k - x)]dx$$
$$+ \int_{t_{k-1}}^{t_k} w(x)[1-Q(t_k - x)]dx, \quad (9.22)$$

for $k = 1,2,\ldots, K$.

As reported by Shen and Zelen[14], the likelihood for women aged t_0 at entry to screening is

$$L(./t_0) = \prod_{k=1}^{K} D_{k,t_0}^{s_{k,t_0}} I_{k,t_0}^{r_{k,t_0}} (1 - D_{k,t_0} - I_{k,t_0})^{n_{k,t_0} - s_{k,t_0} - r_{k,t_0}} \quad (9.23)$$

and the likelihood for the study group is

$$\mathrm{L} = \prod_{t_0=40}^{64} L(./t_0) \quad (9.24)$$

with $K = 4$.

The likelihood Equation (9.24) is revised to include functions for the specificity $\beta(t)$, the transition probability $w(t)dt$, and the probability density $q(.)$ of the sojourn time in S_p. First, suppose the sensitivity at time t is

$$\beta(t) = 1/[1 + \exp(-b_0 - b_1(t - \bar{t}))] \quad (9.25)$$

where $\bar{t}$ is the average age at entry for the study group, and $b_1 > 0$.

Secondly, let the transition function be

$$w(t) = [0.2/\sqrt{2\pi}\sigma t]\exp\{-(\log t - \mu)^2/(2\sigma^2)\}, \quad (9.26)$$

which is the density of a log normal distribution (μ,σ^2). Note that $w(t)dt$ is the transition probability from the disease-free state to the preclinical stage during the time interval t to $t + dt$. According to Ries et al.,[15] the life time risk of being diagnosed with breast cancer is 15.7%, which is less than the lifetime risk of entering the preclinical stage, thus, .20 is a reasonable upper bound. Lastly, for the sojourn time, the survivorship function is

$$Q(x) = 1/[1+(x\rho)^{\kappa}]. \tag{9.27}$$

This form of the sojourn distribution is skewed to the right and has first moment $(\pi/\rho\kappa)\csc(\pi/\kappa)$ and a relatively simple form. This is quite different from Walter and Day[16], who used an exponential distribution.

The Bayesian analysis consists of estimating the six unknown parameters $\theta = (b_0, b_1, \mu, \sigma^2, \kappa, \rho)$ and a prior distribution must be assigned. Consequently, let the prior for (b_0, b_1) be bivariate normal with mean (0,0), and diagonal covariance matrix with diagonal elements 10^{10}. Suppose that $\mu \sim N(0, 10^{10})$ and let the prior for σ^2 be uniform (0,1). For the parameters of the sojourn distribution, suppose that $\kappa \sim uniform(1,5)$ independent of $\rho \sim uniform(0,2)$. A Monte Carlo Markov Chain (MCMC) random sample was generated from the joint posterior distribution using four subchains for $(b_0, b_1); \mu; \sigma^2;$ and (κ, ρ). The MCMC used 30,000 steps with a burn-in of 10,000 iterations. After the burn-in, the posterior was sampled every 20 steps to give a sample of 1000 from the joint posterior distribution. The posterior analysis for the unknown parameters appears in Table 9.16.

Using Equation (9.25) for sensitivity, the posterior mean ranges from .603 to .875 from 40 to 65 years of age, while the posterior standard deviation ranges from .236 to .144 over the same period. The average age of a study participant was 51.6 years, for which the posterior mean sensitivity is .779(.186). This compares closely to Shapiro et al.[17] with a value of .737, computed as the ratio of screen-detected cases divided by the total number of screen and interval detected cases during the 5 years of follow-up.

As for the transition probability from the disease free to the preclinical stage, the posterior medians ranged from $1.388 * 10^{-3}$ at age 40 to $2.735 * 10^{-3}$ at age 65, and the transition function Equation (9.26) appears to peak at age 60.

TABLE 9.16

Posterior Distribution for HIP Study

Parameter	Mean	Median	SD
b_0	1.676	1.581	1.338
b_1	.085	.084	.078
μ	4.340	4.329	.076
σ^2	.190	.172	.076
κ	2.509	2.275	.927
ρ	.886	.917	.287

The average sojourn time was estimated with a posterior mean of 1.88(1.65) and a posterior median of 1.78 years. For more information about the posterior analysis, refer to Wu et al. (Figures 1 and 2 of Reference 9).

How do these results compare to other recent studies? For example, Chen et al.[18] using data from Taiwan, estimated the mean sojourn time as 1.90 years, with a 95% confidence interval from 1.18 to 4.86 years, which compares to a posterior mean estimate of 1.88 years for the present study. However, they modeled the probability distribution as exponential and estimated the sensitivity as 1.

With regard to sensitivity, the present Bayesian estimate varies with age and is the first to present such information. Shen and Zelen[14] assumed a constant sensitivity and estimated it as .70(.20) with a so-called stable model, while it was estimated as .72(.17) with their unstable model. The mean sojourn time was 2.5(1.2) years with the stable model and 2.2(.89) with the unstable, and both estimates are larger than the 1.88 Bayesian estimate.

9.5.2 Bayesian Inference for Lead-Time

The probability distribution for the lead-time is developed for periodic screening examinations. The lead-time is expressed as a mixture of a point mass at zero and a continuous density over the positive numbers. Using the HIP study, simulations are performed to estimate the proportion of breast cancer patients who truly benefit from periodic exams under various screening time intervals. The posterior mean, median, and standard deviation of the lead-time is computed for the various scenarios of screening interval lengths. This information is quite valuable for those who design periodic screening studies.

The difference between the age at diagnosis with mammography and the onset of clinical disease without screening is the lead-time. Suppose the woman enters the preclinical state at time t_1 and becomes clinically incident at time t_2, then $(t_2 - t_1)$ is the sojourn time in the preclinical state. Suppose she is given a mammogram at time t within (t_1, t_2) and cancer is diagnosed, then the lead-time is $t_2 - t$. The distribution of the lead-time depends on the sojourn time, the sensitivity, and the transition probability into the preclinical state. The optimality of a screening program depends very much on the characteristics of the lead-time distribution, hence, good design also depends on the properties of the lead-time.

The lead-time distribution is conditional in that it applies to only those that develop the disease. The typical subject is asymptomatic, will experience a series of screening exams, and will eventually develop breast cancer. Suppose L denotes the lead-time, and that $D = 1$ indicates the presence of breast cancer, otherwise $D = 0$. The lead-time distribution is a mixture of a point mass at zero, $P[L = 0/ D = 1]$, and a conditional density function $f(z/ D = 1)$, where $0 < z < (T - t_0)$ and T is the life span of the subject. In order to compute the lead time distribution, $P[D = 1]$, $P[L = 0, D = 1]$ and the joint density $f(z, D = 1)$ are required. Note that

$$P[D = 1] = \int_{t_0}^{T}\int_{0}^{t} w(x)q(t-x)dxdt \tag{9.28}$$

where w is the transition probability function and q the sojourn time density. The subject is incident with clinical disease at age $t \in (t_0, T)$ and makes the transition from S_0 to S_p at age $x < t$, thus, the sojourn time in the preclinical state is $(t - x)$.

To illustrate the main ideas only two screening exams are considered; consider a group who will have screening exams at ages t_0 and t_1. It can be shown that

$$P[L = 0 , D = 1] = I_{21} + I_{22} \tag{9.29}$$

where

$$I_{21} = [1-\beta(t_0)]\int_{t_0}^{t_1}\int_{0}^{t_0} w(x)q(t-x)dxdt + \int_{t_0}^{t_1}\int_{t_0}^{t} w(x)q(t-x)dxdt. \tag{9.30}$$

I_{21} is the probability of being an interval case in (t_0, t_1), while I_{22} is the probability of being an interval case in (t_1, T), thus

$$\mathrm{I}_{22} = [1-\beta(t_0)][1-\beta(t_1)]\int_{0}^{t_1} w(x)[Q(t_1-x)-Q(T-x)]dx$$

$$+ [1-\beta(t_1)]\int_{t_0}^{t_1} w(x)[Q(t_1-x)-Q(T-x)]dx + \int_{t_1}^{T} w(x)[1-Q(T-x)]dx. \tag{9.31}$$

In a similar way, it can be shown that the joint density is

$$f(z, D = 1) = \beta(t_1)\{(1-\beta(t_0)\int_{0}^{t_0} w(x)q(t_1+z-x)dx + \int_{t_0}^{t_1} w(x)q(t_1+z-x)dx\}$$

$$+\beta(t_0)\int_{0}^{t_0} w(x)q(t_0+z-x)dx \tag{9.32a}$$

and $z \in (0, T - t_1)$.

On the other hand, when $z \in (T - t_1, T - t_0)$,

$$f(z, D = 1) = \beta(t_0) \int_0^{t_0} w(x) q(t_0 + z - x) dx. \tag{9.32b}$$

The screen-detected cases are now considered. Suppose there are K screening exams and let A_j = {a screen detected case at the $(j + 1)$-*st* exam at time t_j} where $j = 0,1,\ldots,K - 1$.

Then, the conditional probability density of the lead-time, given A_j, is

$$f(z/A_j) = f(z, A_j)/P(A_j) \tag{9.33}$$

where

$$f(z, A_j) = \beta_j \left\{ \sum_{i=0}^{j-1} (1-\beta_i)\ldots(1-\beta_{j-1}) \int_{t_{i-1}}^{t_i} w(x) q(t_j + z - x) dx + \int_{t_{j-1}}^{t_j} w(x) q(t_j + z - x) dx \right\} \tag{9.34}$$

and $\beta_i = \beta(t_i)$.

The denominator is

$$P(A_j) = \beta_j \left\{ \sum_{i=0}^{j-1} (1-\beta_i)\ldots(1-\beta_{j-1}) \int_{t_{i-1}}^{t_i} w(x) Q(t_j - x) dx + \int_{t_{j-1}}^{t_j} w(x) Q(t_j - x) dx \right\}. \tag{9.35}$$

All the essential elements have been defined for the computation of the posterior distribution of the lead-time. The lead-time distribution depends on the transition probability function w, the distribution q of the sojourn time, and the time-dependent sensitivity $\beta(t)$, all of which were defined earlier.

The posterior density $f(\theta/data)$, of all the parameters θ, was defined in the previous section and, when it is combined with the conditional lead-time distribution, gives the marginal density

$$\begin{aligned} f(L/\text{data}) &= \int f(L,\theta/data)d\theta = \int f(l/\theta, data) f(\theta/data) d\theta \\ &= \int f(L/\theta) f(\theta/data) d\theta \approx (1/n) \sum_i f(L/\theta_1^*) \end{aligned} \tag{9.36}$$

where θ_i^* is a sample generated from the posterior distribution $f(\theta/data)$. From Equation (9.36) samples of size n can be generated from the posterior

TABLE 9.17

Posterior Distribution of the Lead-time

Interval Months	$P(L = 0)$	Mean	Median	SD	$E(L/L > 0)$
6	.0895	1.418	.50	2.111	1.557
9	.1604	1.282	.38	2.075	1.527
12	.2337	1.168	.30	2.040	1.524
18	.3652	.988	.16	1.969	1.556
24	.4681	.856	.08	1.901	1.605

distribution of the lead-time L. The results from the earlier HIP study are combined with the current model to make inferences about the lead-time for women aged from 50 to 80 years entering a screening program. The results are for both screen-detected and interval cases, allowing inferences for the point mass at zero and the continuous density $f(z/$ data), for $0 < z < 40$. Table 9.17 presents the posterior distribution of L as a function of the time interval between consecutive exams.

Thus, for a woman who begins annual screening at age 40 and continues screenings through age 80, there is a 23% chance that she will not benefit from screening. On the other hand, if she has exams every 6 months, the probability she will benefit is 1–.0895 = .9105. Note that the benefit from screening decreases as the interval between consecutive exams increase, and that the average lead-time also decreases. As the lead-time increases with decreasing interval length between exams, the better the chance of treating the disease earlier.

Of course, there are economic considerations to take into account. More exams per unit time increase the total cost, and the more exams that are scheduled, the chance of missing an exam also increases.

There are two major contributions:

1. The model allows for inference of the lead-time that applies to the total group, both of the screen-detected cases and the interval detected. Earlier contributions such as Prorok[19] included only the screen-detected cases, thus, these results include his as a special case.
2. The model allows for any number of exams and any time interval between consecutive exams. This is a powerful tool for the design of screening trials.

9.6 Decision Theory and Diagnostic Accuracy

What is the impact of a diagnostic test on subsequent care of the patient? Is the most accurate test the most appropriate? In order to answer such questions, a decision theoretic approach can be very useful.

For example, suppose a physician is faced with the following problem: the doctor examines a patient who presents with symptoms indicative of a life threatening disease and surgery is a possibility, but carries a risk of death. There are three possibilities: (1) do nothing, (2) perform surgery, or (3) order an imaging test, and proceed accordingly. If nothing is done, the patient avoids the risk of death by surgery. If the chance of having the disease is high, surgery is appropriate if the risk of death by surgery is less than the risk of having the disease. Finally an imaging test can be ordered and, if negative, nothing is done, but if positive surgery is in order. Which of the three alternatives should be taken?

Decision theory can be used here if one has additional information. One would need to know the probability of having the disease, the probability of disease, if the test is positive, the probability of no disease if the test is negative, the sensitivity and the specificity, and the chance of dying by surgery.

Finally, one would need to know the life expectancy of the patient for the following scenarios:

1. Do nothing
   a. When the disease is present
   b. When disease it is not there

2. Surgery
   a. When the disease is present and death by surgery
   b. When the disease is present and no death by surgery
   c. When the disease is not present and there is death by surgery
   d. When the disease is not present and there is no death by surgery

3. Imaging

   a. When the test is positive, the disease is present, and death by surgery
   b. When the test is positive, the disease is present, and no death by surgery
   c. When the test is positive, the disease is not present, and there is death due to surgery
   d. When the test is positive, the disease is not present, and there is no death due to surgery
   e. The test is negative and there is disease
   f. The test is negative and there is no disease

Therefore, the life expectancy must be specified for 10 scenarios, 2 for when nothing is done, 4 when surgery is performed, and 6 under the imaging alternative.

TABLE 9.18

Lifetime for Three Alternatives

Option	Lifetime
Do Nothing	$P(D+)L_1 + P(D-)L_2$
Surgery	$P(D+)[P(S+)L_3 + P(S-)L_4] + P(D-)[P(S+)L_5 + P(S-)L_6]$
Imaging	$P(T+)\{P(D+/T+)[P(S+)L_7 + P(S-)L_8]$
	$+ P(D-/T+)[P(S+)L_9 + P(S-)L_{10}]\}$
	$+ P(T+)[P(D+/T-)L_{11} + P(D-/T-)L_{12}]$

Although decision theory can be helpful, one is faced with having to find 14 probabilities and 12 life expectancies. Where is such information found? Once the information becomes available, the life expectancy under the three alternatives can be computed, and the optimal alternative selected by choosing the one with the smallest overall average life expectancy. This is summarized in Table 9.18. (See Plevritis[20] [Figure 1].)

For example, L_1 is the patient's lifetime when the disease is present ($D+$), while L_3 is the lifetime when the disease is present and there is death due to surgery ($S+$). For the third alternative, L_7 is the lifetime when the imaging test is positive ($T+$), the disease is present, and there is death due to surgery, etc.

One must find the values for the probabilities and average lifetimes. This was done by Plevritis in an excellent introduction to decision making for radiologists. These values are used in this presentation as follows. The probabilities are represented as beta(a,b) random variables where the probabilities are given by Plevritis. The probability is given by $a/(a+b)$, where $a+b$ is the number of patients having the given probability, and the $a+b$ values are varied to reflect various levels of confidence in the probability values. The lifetime is assumed to be an exponential random variable, where the life expectancies are given in Table 2 of Plevritis. Once these are given, the average life expectancy under the three scenarios can be computed and the one with the smallest value selected as the optimal choice of treatment.

For example, the average value of $P(D+)L_1 + P(D-)L_2$ is computed, assuming $P(D+) \sim$ beta(1,9), L_1 as exponential with mean 65, and L_2 as exponential with mean 80 years; therefore, under the "do nothing" alternative, the life expectancy is .1(65) + .9(80) = 78.5 years, assuming the two lifetimes are independent. Note, that by assuming $P(D+) \sim$ beta(1,9), one is assuming there are 10 patients, one of which has disease. By varying $a+b$, one varies the posterior standard deviation of the overall expected lifetime. It is interesting how the test accuracy enters the computation for the average lifetime for the test imaging alternative. For additional information on the decision theory approach to diagnostic medicine, see Parmigiami[21].

9.7 Exercises

9.1 Refer to Table 9.1 and Table 9.2. (a) Suppose the prevalence of breast cancer among those eligible for the present study (say, from ages 35 to 60) is .05., then what is the posterior distribution of the TPF and the FPF? (b) Is there a lower positive limit on the prevalence rate? If so, estimate it.

9.2 (a) Verify Table 9.4 and compute the 95% credible interval for each parameter, and test the hypothesis that TPF for mammography is greater than that for MRI. (b) Perform the posterior analysis of the correlation between the detection probabilities of the two modalities.

9.3 Using Minitab, estimate the DP and FRP. (See Table 9.5.)

9.4 Referring to Table 9.5, the main hypothesis is that the $DP_{ct} > DP_{x-ray}$. Are the sample sizes sufficient? What are the implications for the TPF of CT vs. X-ray?

9.5 The breast cancer screening trial with mammography and MRI was paired, then compared to an unpaired layout for the national lung cancer screening trial. Describe the advantages and disadvantages of paired vs. unpaired designs.

9.6 If a subset of the test negative subjects are subject to the gold standard, show that the TPF and FPF are biased upwards.

9.7 Show that Equation (9.7) follows from Bayes theorem.

9.8 Verify the posterior analysis of Table 9.8 and compare the 95% credible interval for the Bayesian analysis with the 95% confidence interval for the TPF using result 7.4 of Pepe.[6] Also find the posterior mean, standard deviation, and the 95% credible interval for the FPF.

9.9 Employing a uniform prior distribution for the four gamma parameters of Table 9.9, find the posterior distribution of the TPF. Use Minitab or WinBUGS to generate observations from the joint posterior distribution of the parameters. Are the posterior mean and standard deviation the same as those of Table 9.8? If not, explain why? Of the two analyses (based on Table 9.7 and Table 9.9), which are the most appropriate and which are the most misleading? Explain your answers in detail.

9.10 The prior information for the stool exam parameters are $s_1 \sim$ beta(4.44,13.31) and $c_1 \sim$ beta(71.25,3.75) (see Joseph et al.[7](p. 266)), and when combined with the prior information for serology (see Equation (9.9)) and the likelihood function Equation 9.10, the joint posterior distribution is determined. Write a WinBUGS program and perform the posterior analysis for the sensitivity and specificity of both diagnostic tests and disease prevalence. Refer to the appendix of the Joseph article.

9.11 (a) Verify Table 9.15. (b) Test the hypothesis H: $\gamma \le 1$ vs. A: $\gamma > 1$. Is iNOS highly associated with survival? (c) Is the sample size sufficient for testing H vs. A?

9.12 Extend the measure of association γ Equation (9.14) between a diagnostic test and survival to include more than two ordinal diagnostic scores.

9.13 Refer to formulas Equation (9.15) to Equation (9.18) and Obuchowski.[2] (a) With the Bayesian approach, estimate the ROC area of the percent transferrin saturation, assuming a uniform prior for the ROC area. (b) Write a WinBUGS program that compares the ROC areas of the two diagnostic tests. Do not ignore the correlation between the two areas.

9.14 (a) Refer to Wu et al.[9] and verify Figure 1 using formulas Equation (9.25) and Equation (9.26) above. (b) From Table 9.16, is there evidence that age affects the sensitivity? Test the relevant hypothesis. (c) How well does the model fit the data? Describe the relevant goodness of fit tests for adequacy of the Bayesian model.

9.15 From the literature, find other screening programs (heart disease and lung cancer) and apply the concepts above to describe the transition probability from the disease-free state to the preclinical state, the distribution of the sojourn time in the preclinical state, and the time-dependent sensitivity function of the screening method (e.g., CT for lung cancer).

9.16 (a) Refer to Table 9.18 of Section 9.6 and write a WinBUGS program to compute the average lifetime and the corresponding standard deviations of the three alternatives. Assume the probabilities are beta random variables and the lifetimes are exponentially distributed. Assume the appropriate random variables are independent. (b) What alternative gives the smallest life expectancy? The smallest standard deviation?

References

1. Ekmekcioglu, S., Ellerhorst, J.A., Prieto, V.G., Johnson, M.M., Broemeling, L.D., Grimm, E.A., Tumor iNOS predicts poor survival for stage III melanoma patients, *Int. J. Cancer,* 15, 119, 861, 2006.
2. Obuchowski, N.A., Estimating and comparing diagnostic tests' accuracy when the gold standard is not binary, *Acad. Radiol.*, 12, 1198, 2005.
3. Obuchowski, N.A., An ROC type measure of diagnostic accuracy when the gold standard is continuous scale, *Stat. Med.*, 25, 481, 2005.
4. Moore, S.M, Gierada, D.S., Clark, K.W., Blaine, G.J., and the PLCO-NLST Quality Assurance Working Group, Image quality assurance in prostate, lung, colorectal, and ovarian cancer screening trial network of the national lung screening program, *J. Digit. Imag.*, 18, 242, 2005.
5. Begg, C.B. and Greenes, R.A., Assessment on diagnostic tests when disease verification is subject to selection bias, *Biometrics,* 39, 207, 1983.

6. Pepe, M.S., *The Statistical Evaluation of Medical Tests for Classification and Prediction*, Oxford University Press, 2003, Oxford, U.K.
7. Joseph, L., Gyorkis, T.W., and Coupal, L., Bayesian estimation of disease prevalence and the parameters of diagnostic tests in the absence of a gold standard, *Am. J. Epidemiol.*, 141, 263, 1995.
8. Pencina, M.J. and D'Agostino, R.B., Overall C as a measure of discrimination in survival analysis: model, specific population value, and confidence interval estimation, *Stat. Med.*, 23, 2109, 2004.
9. Wu, D., Rosner, G., and Broemeling, L.D. MLE and Bayesian inference of age-dependent sensitivity and transition probability in periodic screening, *Biometrics*, 61, 1056, 2005.
10. Wu, D., Rosner, G., and Broemeling, L.D., Bayesian inference for the lead-time in periodic cancer screening, *Biometrics*, 2006, in press.
11. Berry, D.A., Cronin, K.A., Plevritie, S.K., Fryback, D.G., Clar, L., Zelen, M., Mandelblatt, J.S., Yakolev, A.Y., Habbema, J.D.F., and Feuer, E., Effect of screening and adjuvant therapy on mortality from breast cancer, *N. Engl. J. Med.*, 353, 1784, 2005.
12. Zelen, M., Optimal scheduling of examinations for the early detection of disease. *Biometrics*, 80, 279, 1993.
13. Lee, S.J. and Zelen, M., Scheduling periodic examinations for the early detection of disease: applications to breast cancer, *J. Am. Stat. Assoc.*, 93, 1271, 1999.
14. Shen, Y., and Zelen, M., Parametric estimation procedures for screening programs: stable and nonstable disease models for multimodality case finding, *Biometrics*, 86, 503, 1999.
15. Ries, L.A.G., Eisner, M.P., Kosary, C.L., Hankey, P.F., Miller, A.B., Clegg , L., and Edwards, B.K., SEER cancer statistics review, 1973–1999, Bethesda, MD: National Cancer Institute, 2002, Available at: http//seer.cancer.gov/csr/1973-1999/.
16. Walter, S.D. and Day, N.E., Estimation of the duration of a preclinical disease using screening data, *Am. J. Epidemiol.*, 118, 856, 1983.
17. Shapiro, S., Venet, W., Strax, P., and Venet, L., *Periodic Screening for Breast Cancer. The Health Insurance Plan Project and its Sequelae, 1963-1986*, The Johns Hopkins University Press, 1988, Baltimore, MD.
18. Chen, T.H.H., Kuo, H.S., Yen, M.F., Lai, M.S., Tabar, L., and Duffy, S.W., Estimation of sojourn time in chronic disease screening data on interval cases. *Biometrics*, 56, 167, 2000.
19. Prorok, P.C., Bounded recurrence times and lead-time in the design of a repetitive screening program, *J. Appl. Probab.*, 19, 10, 1982.
20. Plevritis, S.K., Decision analysis and simulation modeling for evaluating diagnostic tests on the basis of patients outcomes, *Am. J. Radiol.*, 185, 581, 2005.
21. Parmigiani, G., *Modeling in Medical Decision Making: a Bayesian Approach*, John Wiley & Sons, 2002, New York.

Index

A

B

I

L

M

N

P

Q

R

S

T

V

W